Promoting Children's Emotional Well-being

Messages from Research

Edited by

Ann Buchanan and Barbara L. Hudson

*Department of Social Policy and Social Work,
University of Oxford*

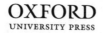

OXFORD
UNIVERSITY PRESS

OXFORD
UNIVERSITY PRESS

Great Clarendon Street, Oxford OX2 6DP

Oxford University Press is a department of the University of Oxford.
It furthers the University's objective of excellence in research, scholarship,
and education by publishing worldwide in

Oxford New York

Athens Auckland Bangkok Bogotá Buenos Aires Calcutta
Cape Town Chennai Dar es Salaam Delhi Florence Hong Kong Istanbul
Karachi Kuala Lumpur Madrid Melbourne Mexico City Mumbai
Nairobi Paris São Paulo Singapore Taipei Tokyo Toronto Warsaw

with associated companies in
Berlin Ibadan

Oxford is a registered trade mark of Oxford University Press
in the UK and in certain other countries

Published in the United States
by Oxford University Press Inc., New York

© Oxford University Press, 2000

A catalogue record for this book is available from the British Library

British Library Cataloguing in Publication Data
Data available

Library of Congress Cataloging in Publication Data
1 3 5 7 9 10 8 6 4 2

ISBN 0 19 263174 8

Typeset by Phoenix Photosetting, Chatham, Kent
Printed in Great Britain on acid free paper by
Biddles Ltd, Guildford & King's Lynn

Promoting Children's Emotional Well-being

Preface

What is emotional well-being in children? Why should we be concerned about promoting it? What part does parenting play in children's psychological health? What role have schools, the legal system, and the wider social environment?

Is promoting emotional well-being in children just the reverse of preventing maladjustment, or is it more than that—the X factor that helps children develop into happier, more satisfied, more achieving, more responsible citizens of tomorrow?

This book, written by leading researchers, many of whom are at the cutting edge of their subject, explores some of these complex interrelationships. It brings together some of the most recent research messages from health, education, psychology, socio-legal, and social studies, and the young people themselves.

This book comes at a time when there is concern about the growing numbers of children with emotional and behavioural difficulties; difficulties that affect their educational progress in school, relationships with their parents and in turn their relationships with peers, partners, and adult psychological and physical health.

Children with emotional and behavioural problems are by the very nature of their difficulties, in the current UK Government jargon, 'socially excluded'. These children are part of our 'social capital' of tomorrow. What can be done to ensure that all children are socially 'included'?

This is the second book from the *Centre for Research into Parenting and Children*, Oxford University. (The first book, also a collection of research findings, *Parenting, Schooling and Children's Behaviour* was published by Ashgate in 1998). The specific aims of the Centre are:

- To develop a better understanding of the well-being of parents and children; what causes problems (health, education, psychological, and social) and how they may be ameliorated.
- To build interdisciplinary research links.
- To act as a forum for discussion for researchers from different disciplines and for practitioners (health, education, psychological, and social) who work with children and families.
- To disseminate research findings.

The current members are:

Dr Ann Buchanan: University Lecturer in Applied Social Studies, Department of Social Policy and Social Work

Professor Kathy Sylva: Professor of Educational Psychology, Department of Educational Studies

Dr Catherine Baillie: Chartered Psychologist, Department of Educational Studies

Dr Sarah Stewart-Brown: Director of the Health Services Research Unit, Department of Public Health

Dr Jane Barlow: MRC Research Fellow at the Health Services Research Unit, Department of Public Health

Dr Jane Wells: Consultant in Public Health Medicine, Berkshire Health Authority and an Associate Member, Health Services Research Unit, Department of Public Health

Dr Frances Gardner: Clinical Psychologist and University Lecturer in Applied Social Studies, Department of Social Policy and Social Work

Mrs Teresa Smith: Director of the Department of Social Policy and Social Work

Mavis Maclean: Senior Research Fellow, Centre for Socio-Legal Studies, Wolfson College

Joan Hunt: Senior Research Fellow, Centre for Socio-Legal Studies, Wolfson College

Ann Buchanan and Barbara L. Hudson

Oxford
September 2000

Contents

Contributors

Catherine Baillie, BA Hons (University of Liverpool), PhD (University of Leeds)
Catherine Baillie is a chartered psychologist. Her doctoral research investigated the psychological sequelae of genetic testing in pregnancy. She went on to coordinate a national psychosocial study of predictive testing for breast cancer predisposition genes. She now coordinates a longitudinal study of the effects of different forms of childcare on child development, at the Department of Educational Studies, University of Oxford.

Victoria Bream, BA (Oxon)
Victoria Bream studied at Oxford University, gaining a degree in experimental psychology. She is currently a research assistant at the Department of Social Policy and Social Work, University of Oxford, and is working on a number of projects linked to the Centre for Research into Parenting and Children. The main focus of her present work is with Ann Buchanan, Joan Hunt, and others on a Nuffield Foundation Project accessing parents' and children's perspectives on welfare reporting under Section 8 of the Children Act 1989.

Ann Buchanan, PhD (Southampton) MA (Oxon), CQSW
Ann Buchanan is University Lecturer in Applied Social Studies and a Fellow of St Hilda's College, Oxford. Before entering academic life in 1990, she spent ten years working as a child psychiatric social worker in an inner urban area. Her current research interests are the consequences of emotional and behavioural problems in children, and long-term outcomes. Some of her research, as in this volume, is based on secondary analysis of longitudinal studies, but her work is informed by surveys of

young people's views and field studies of parents' and children's perspectives.

Recent research grants have come from The Nuffield Foundation, NHS Executive (Anglia and Oxon), Joseph Rowntree Foundation, The Mental Health Foundation, The Samaritans, and Barnardo's.

Deborah M. Capaldi, BA (University of York, England), PhD (University of Oregon, USA)

Deborah Capaldi is a research scientist at the Oregon Social Learning Center and principal investigator on the Oregon Youth Study. Her work centres on the causes and consequences of anti-social behaviour across the life span, including aggression in young couples' relationships, health-risking sexual behaviours, and intergenerational transmission of risk.

J. Mark Eddy, PhD

Mark Eddy is a research scientist at the NIMH-funded Oregon Prevention Research Center, part of the Oregon Social Learning Center (*www.oslc.org*) in Eugene. His research focuses on the development and refinement of interventions to prevent parent and child problem behaviours. He is currently the principal investigator of the Paths Project, which is examining the transition to young adulthood for serious juvenile offenders.

Emma Evans, BA (Hons) Psychology

Emma Evans is a research assistant at the Department of Psychiatry, University of Oxford. Previously she worked under Professor Sylva as a research assistant on *Effective Provision of Preschool Education*, a project funded by the Department of Education and Employment.

Eirini Flouri, BSc, PhD

Eirini Flouri holds a degree in psychology from the University of Crete, Greece, and a PhD in psychology from Exeter University. She has worked as a research officer in the Refugee Studies Centre at Queen Elizabeth House at Oxford University and is currently a research assistant at the Department of Social Policy and Social Work, working with Ann Buchanan. She has published in the areas of economic psychology and especially economic socialisation and consumer values. Her current interests are children's resiliency and recovery from emotional and behavioural problems.

Frances Gardner, MA, MPhil, DPhil
Frances Gardner is currently University Lecturer in Applied Social Studies in the Department of Social Policy and Social Work. Previously she was University Lecturer in Clinical Psychology at the University Department of Psychiatry, Park Hospital in Oxford. Before that, she was Lecturer at the Institute of Psychiatry and Senior Clinical Psychologist at the Maudesley Hospital working with families in Camberwell. She was also Lecturer in Education at Warwick University. Her current research interests include a randomised trial of parenting programmes and a Wellcome-funded longitudinal observational study of parenting style and the early development of children's behaviour problems. Other grants include co-investigator on the MRC Hip Trial, investigating the psychosocial effects on parents of babies with hip instability. She is a member of the Steering Committee of the DoH ECMO Trial advising about the measurement of psychological outcomes in children with neonatal respiratory illness. She is co-editor of the 'Measurement Issues' series in *Child Psychology and Psychiatry Review*.

Roger Grimshaw, MA (Cantab), PhD (Birmingham)
Roger Grimshaw is Research Director of the Centre for Crime and Justice Studies, King's College, London. Its research programme is developing a significant theme around services for young people in custody. He has lectured in both education and criminology and has published widely in the field of vulnerable and challenging young people. He was formerly Senior Research Officer at the National Children's Bureau, and responsible for a variety of projects. His work on the review of children's care plans helped produce conclusions that were published as part of a report by a parliamentary select committee.

Barbara L. Hudson, MA (Cantab), CQSW
Barbara Hudson is University Lecturer in Applied Social Studies

at the University Department of Social Policy and Social Work. She was previously at the London School of Economics and, before that, a psychiatric social worker. A former editor of the *British Journal of Social Work*, she has also co-edited a series of psychiatry texts. Her main interests are cognitive–behavioural approaches in social work and the development of evidence-based social work.

Joan Hunt, MA (Cantab) Dip. Social Administration; Home Office Certificate of Recognition in Child Care
Joan Hunt is a senior research fellow at the University of Oxford's Centre for Socio-Legal Studies. She trained and practised as a social worker before becoming an academic researcher in 1985. She has researched extensively in the area of children's law, focusing on the operation of the family justice system and its interface with the family and social welfare institutions.

Adrienne Katz, BA (Rand)
Adrienne Katz is founder of the registered charity Young Voice, which listens and responds to young people. In this capacity she serves as a member of the Learning for Life steering group of the Work/Life Forum, the Boys' working group at the Sex Education Forum at the National Children's Bureau, and as a consultant to Reach for the Sky, a careers advice programme. Her work as an author and journalist has included several books for parents and a study of working mothers (*The juggling act*, 1992, Bloomsbury). Her writing has covered family issues, the child's viewpoint, and tension between paid work and parenting. She writes for a number of newspapers and magazines. In 1995, Adrienne Katz carried out Family Values, a national survey of family life supported by Sainsbury's and Exploring Parenthood as a contribution toward the International Year of the Family. Social research projects have been devised and undertaken since 1996 with Ann Buchanan which aim to communicate the findings of research to a wide audience of youth workers, parents, teachers, health workers, policy makers, and young people. Recent work within this partnership has been carried out for The Samaritans and The Mental Health Foundation in addition to Young Voice projects.

Sarah Stewart-Brown, FRCP, FFPHM, PhD (Bristol), MA, BM, BCh (Oxon)
Sarah Stewart-Brown is Director of the Health Services Research Unit in the Department of Public Health. Her past research has been mainly in two fields, community child health and health promotion. Her current research interest covers the importance of emotional well-being for public health and the particular importance of emotional health in childhood for both mental and physical health in adulthood. She is carrying out research on the impact of parenting on health and on the effectiveness of parenting programmes and emotional literacy programmes in schools.

Kathy Sylva, PhD (Harvard)
Kathy Sylva is Professor of Educational Psychology at the Department of Educational Studies, University of Oxford. She is an international authority on early education and currently co-director of large scale research projects investigating effective provision of pre-school education, the effects of child care on child development; she is also evaluating a community programme aimed at supporting parents in the management of their children's behaviour and learning.

Sarah Ward, BSc (Hons) (Bristol)
Sarah Ward is a clinical psychologist in training at the Warneford Hospital, Oxford. In 1996 she was awarded a Medical Research Council studentship to carry out DPhil research on parenting, conscience, and children's conduct problems in the University Department of Psychiatry, based at the Park Hospital for Children. Previously she worked in Yorkshire as an assistant psychologist in community mental health for the elderly and in health psychology at Leeds University.

Jane Wells, MFPHM, MSc, MB, BCh
Jane Wells is Consultant in Public Health Medicine, Berkshire Health Authority; and an associate member, Health Services Research Unit, Department of Public Health, University of Oxford. Until 31 October 1999 she was Senior Registrar in Public Health Medicine at the Health Services Research Unit. She

is a public health physician who has previously worked as a junior hospital doctor and in general practice and community child health in the UK. She has also carried out research in West Africa and spent some time at the Baltimore Cochrane Center, USA, part of the international Cochrane Collaboration. Her interests include child health and health promotion, particularly the promotion of children's mental health and prevention of emotional and behaviour problems. She is also interested in the evaluation and implementation of health promoting and health care interventions, and the presentation of health-related information in the media.

1

Present issues and concerns

___

Ann Buchanan

'If we are to improve the lives of children . . . we must face the reality that the human infant and young child is incapable of autonomous self-protective behaviour. . . . the human species gives birth to offspring that experience years of physical, emotional and mental development almost entirely controlled and influenced by significant adults responsible for nurturance and care. While maturational processes are built into the developing organism, each of these processes requires a nutritious diet, physical care, social stimulation and consistent parenting' **Albee 1992, p. 327**

'As we approach the millennium it is appropriate that we consider what we have learned from psychosocial risk research and what are the challenges ahead that must be met. . . . the dismissal of environmental influences by genetic evangelists is not justified. The rise over time during the last 50 years in the rates of many disorders in young people makes it clear that environmental factors of some kind must be influential.' **Rutter 1999a, p. 490**

This book is about promoting the emotional well-being of a vulnerable developing organism – the human infant. It is about strategies that assist children to maximise their potential and increase the quality of their lives as they mature into adulthood and autonomy. Inevitably this book is also about the other side of the coin: the prevention of emotional and behavioural disorders that affect a child's relationships with their family and others, inhibit their progress in school, and are associated with a range of problems in adult life.

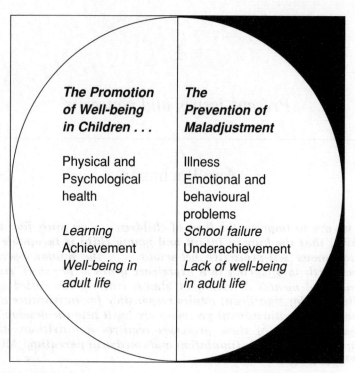

Fig.1.1 The relationship between well-being and the prevention of maladjustment.

A more comprehensive discussion on the concept of 'well-being' is given in Chapter 2, but an underlying assumption in this book is that any activity or service that promotes a child's development, adaptation or functioning has the reciprocal benefit of preventing maladjustment, delay or disorder (Simeonsson 1994).

Is maladjustment preventable?

Allied to this is a second assumption: that the manifestation of problems or conditions associated with maladjustment is largely preventable. Until recently few would have questioned this assumption. Albee (1992), for example, would argue that if we are to improve the well-being of children, we must improve the environment of the developing child. It was only a question of finding out how best to do this. The arrival of strong findings, however, from the behavioural genetic researchers has removed some of this certainty. 'When it comes to a child's emotional well-being, it is all in their genes.' If this is true, psychosocial interventions have a limited role.

Behavioural geneticists have expressed scepticism about the importance of psychosocial influences except at the extremes (Scarr 1992, Rowe 1994). Albee, they may say, is talking about children 'living on the brink' where the extremes of poverty seriously impinge on children's lives. Most children in the developed world do not live in such extreme conditions and so most children do all right regardless of their environment.

Children's genes, they also say, influence the life they lead. Plomin and Bergeman (1991), for example, demonstrate that individual differences have been shown to influence exposure to psychosocial risk – would John Kennedy have died in his aeroplane had risk-taking not been in his genes? Further, Plomin and Daniels (1987) argue that psychological traits, rather than the way children are treated, explain why children in the same family are so different. Scarr (1997) has gone so far as to propose that 'genetic theory' should replace 'socialisation theory'.

Rutter (1999a) claims that despite these strong findings there are good grounds for acknowledging the psychosocial influences on childhood.

Central to Rutter's argument is evidence of a huge rise in psychosocial disorders among young people over the last fifty years (Rutter and Smith 1995) which he feels must be related to environmental factors. It is implausible, he contends, that in such a short space of time the genetic pool could have changed so rapidly. It has become increasingly clear in the nature/nurture debate that even in strongly genetic psychological disorders, environmental factors play a substantial role, not only in the aetiology, but also in the maintenance or otherwise of the disorder.

The focus needs to shift from the precipitants of the onset of disorder to an understanding of the processes that operate over time in the

initiation and course of disorders as they remit and relapse. The importance of indirect chain reactions is obvious but much has still to be
learned about how they operate. ... How do they bring about the
effects and what determines whether the effects persist or fade? More
than anything else this last question requires that psychosocial
research be part of biological psychiatry. In looking to the future it is to
be hoped that the absurd dualisms of the past can be put behind us.
(Rutter 1999a, p. 490)

If then, there is a role for promoting psychological well-being,
a final assumption is that the best time to 'prevent' problems is
sooner rather than later. As Simeonsson (1994) notes, we need
to capitalise on the momentum provided by the developmental
forces in childhood. This is not so much because early experiences inevitably shape later behaviour but rather, as shown by
more recent longitudinal research, that events in early childhood
can set off an indirect chain reaction that seriously interferes
with life chances (Rutter and Smith 1995).

Why does emotional well-being in children matter?

At different times in history, there have been very different views
about childhood. 'Childhood', as distinct from infancy, adolescence or young adulthood, was unknown in historical times.
Young boys dressed as little versions of their fathers, they played
as their fathers 'and were hung by their necks' like their fathers
(Illich 1973). Stainton Rogers (1989) argues that the fact that we
no longer burn children as witches or brand them as vagrants is not
the work of the social reformers, it is the result of a whole society
constructing a new social reality about children and childhood. In
essence, every modern society has a moral responsibility to
ensure, as far as possible, the well-being of their children.
Children in most parts of the world today have rights framed by
the UN Convention, 1989 and encoded in national legislation. In
England and Wales, for instance, under the Children Act, 1989:

When a court determines any question with respect to the upbringing
of a child . . .
The child's welfare shall be the court's paramount consideration . . .
(Section 1)

The court shall have particular regard to: . . . his physical, emotional and educational needs. (Section 4(b))

Links between behavioural problems in childhood, delinquency and adult offending

Apart from the legal duty, there are sound socio-political reasons for ensuring children's emotional and behavioural adjustment. Research by Farrington (1988) and Robins (1986), among others, has consistently found that a constellation of childhood antisocial behaviour predicts a constellation of adult antisocial behaviour. Numerous studies from different parts of the world have shown that childhood conduct problems predict later offending (e.g. Loeber and LeBlanc 1990). Spivack *et al.* (1986) in Philadelphia demonstrated that troublesome kindergarten behaviour as early as age 3 and 4 predicted later police contacts. Similarly, in Montreal, ratings of aggressiveness by teachers and peers at ages 6 and 7 predicted self-reported offending at ages 14 to 15 (Tremblay *et al.* 1988).

A further concern is that there are considerable links between juvenile and adult offending. Robins (1986) has shown that whilst no more than half of conduct-disordered children became antisocial adults, virtually all antisocial adults had previously shown symptoms of conduct disorder as children. In the UK, the Home Office, the ministry responsible for crime and disorder, is taking an increasing interest in children who are presenting with behavioural problems. Indeed, the green paper with proposals for *'Supporting Families'* came not from the Department of Health which is the ministry more usually concerned with family issues, but from the Home Office (Home Office 1998). The implication is that supporting families and improving parenting are central to strategies for reducing crime.

There are other concerns associated with children with behavioural problems. As more and more children and young people in the UK move through education achieving more examination successes (Department of Education and Employment 1999), at the other end of the scale, more children are being suspended from school for disruptive behaviour (Cabinet Office, Social Exclusion Unit 1998). School offers children the best chance for redressing early life disadvantages. In the UK, as schools compete

for the best pupils by publishing the results of children's achievement tests, there is less tolerance for children who disrupt others'
education. Expulsion from school is like handing a child a free
ticket to delinquency. Quite apart from the tragedy this causes in
the child's life, society loses out on what the young person could
have contributed economically had he/she remained in school.
Society also has to pay the cost of welfare benefits if the young
person later cannot find work.

*Links between emotional disorders in childhood, depression in
adulthood and major physical illness*

Children with emotional disorders, that is those with anxiety and
depression, are also of concern, in that they are more likely to
present with mental health problems in adult life than those
without such disorders. Kovacs and Devlin (1998) note that
findings from epidemiological, community-based and clinical
referred samples have shown a continuity from anxiety and
depression in childhood into adolescence and from adolescence
into young adulthood.

   More recently, as Stewart-Brown will demonstrate in chapter
two, a further major concern is evidence that there are links
between psychological disorders in childhood/adulthood and
major physical illness in adult life. Children's emotional well-
being has become a major public health issue.

Intergenerational links

A final concern is that the children with emotional and behavioural problems, in their turn, become the parents of the next
generation. Parenting at the best of times is challenging. It is particularly so for those who are also trying to live on a low income
with their own mental health problems (Buchanan 1996).

**Causes of maladjustment – key influences from research
over the last fifty years**

Over the past fifty years, theories on the causation of psychological disorders have abounded. At times the debate has been

In childhood
➢ Poorer family relationships
➢ Lower levels of school achievement
➢ Greater risk of school suspension/expulsion
➢ Links with offending behaviour
➢ Fewer qualifications
➢ Poorer employment prospects
➢ Social exclusion

In adult life
➢ Links with mental health problems
➢ Possible links with a range of serious physical illnesses

Intergenerational links
➢ Poorer relationships with partners and own children
➢ Possible problems in parenting
➢ Another generation of children with their own problems

Buchanan (1999). *What works for troubled children*

Fig. 1.2 Some possible consequences of emotional and behavioural problems.

fierce. Looking back over our history, apparently opposing theoretical stances are not as contradictory as they once appeared. As new findings presented, some pieces of the jigsaw fitted and some had to be discarded, but overall most influences have contributed to the knowledge base we have today.

Current views on emotional well-being – the ecological framework

As research evidence grew, it became apparent that although the interactions of the child with his/her parents were central to the child's psychological well-being, the child and his/her family operated in a social context which also influenced their mental health. Faced with the complexity of research findings many practitioners and researchers turned to the ecological model (Bronfenbrenner 1979) as a convenient framework to incorpo-

Table 1.1 What causes psychological disorders in children? Review of research in the last fifty years.

Some key influences	Implications	Current view	Some key studies
Situation in 1948			
Mental hygiene movement	Interpersonal relationships at home and at school shaped children's behaviour.	Still relevant.	Hewitt and Jenkins 1946
Psychoanalysis	Intra-psychic mental mechanisms/ past experiences and maladaptive parent/child relationships shaped behaviour.	Some of the more extreme ideas such as the 'refrigerator parent' causing autism have been disproved.	Baldwin 1968; Dare 1976
Developmental studies	Early studies, e.g. of foster children, concluded that part of what appeared to be an environmental influence on mental development was actually genetically mediated.	Although some of the methodologies may appear crude by present-day standards, the quality of much of the work was high.	Leahy 1935 (children in foster care). Skeels and Dye 1939 experimental study to improve conditions in residential care.
Behaviourism	Children's behaviour was influenced, and could be modified by, social learning approaches.	Among the most effective treatment approaches— especially cognitive/behavioural.	Skinner, 1938; Miller and Dollard 1941

1950s and early 1960s

Role of maternal deprivation	Strong claims were made re. the supposedly severely damaging, pervasive and irreversible effects of even short separations of a child from its mother.	Empirical research findings have indicated that the damage was not as inevitable or as irreversible as first thought. 'Internal working models' may be important.	Bowlby 1951; Critique by Wootton 1959; Current research: Van Ijzendoorn 1995
Learning from animal studies	Animal studies were consistent in showing that early experiences could have important lasting effects. e.g. Harlow's monkeys, Levine's rats.	Most studies dealt with extreme environmental conditions.	Harlow 1958; Levine 1962
Role of peer relationships	Study demonstrated the importance of peer relationships in promoting resilience.	Ongoing relevance.	Freud and Dann 1951
Role of social groups	Bandura's experimental studies of imitation.	Other work showed it was important to focus on social context in which the groups operated; e.g. school.	Bandura and Walters 1963; Barker and Wright 1955

1960 and 1970s

Child effect on parents	The New York longitudinal study pointed to the importance of children's temperamental characteristics.	Many of the effects attributed to parents may actually be the other way around.	Thomas et al. 1968

Table 1.1 – *continued*

Some key influences	Implications	Current view	Some key studies
1960 and 1970s – *continued*			
Risk indicators and risk mechanisms	Rutter's work in the Isle of Wight and that of the cohort studies showed that quite detailed measures of psychosocial risk factors could be established.	Care is needed to separate risk indicators from mechanisms. With the broadening of risk research, findings show the importance of conflict, rivalries, insecurities and individual differences.	Rutter *et al.* 1970
Role of schooling	Rutter's study showed substantial school effects on both pupil behaviour and scholastic attainments.	This was confirmed by subsequent research	Rutter *et al.* 1979; Maughan 1994 Mortimore 1995
Effects of residential care	Children's behaviour was influenced by the characteristics of institutions providing substitute parental care.	In recent years evidence has emerged showing that the 'care' experience may not improve children's well-being	Tizard *et al.* 1975; Cheung and Buchanan 1997
The influence of area/community	Rutter's comparison between the Isle of Wight and a borough in inner London confirmed that there were important area influences.	More recent studies demonstrate that there are true area or community effects independent of family characteristics.	Rutter and Quinton 1977; Macintyre and Ellaway 1999

The effects of adverse life events	In adults the emphasis was on acute life events and the timing of the onset of disorder while with children the focus was more on the effects of chronic psychosocial adversities.	Today psychological disorders are felt to be more associated with multiple adversities rather than a single acute life event. Timing of disorder is probably less significant.	Brown and Harris 1978

1980s and early 1990s

Indirect long-term effects; Vulnerability factors; Distal and proximal factors.	Reviews at the beginning of the 1980s, e.g. Clarke and Clarke, concluded that there were few serious long-term sequelae to adverse early life events. It was later shown long-term sequelae did arise through *indirect chain effects* making the child more vulnerable to later adversities.	The debate remains about the mechanisms; e.g. is it poverty per se, or the indirect effects of parenting which is harder when living in poverty? 'parents need permissive circumstances in which to parent.'	Clarke and Clarke 1976; Conger *et al.* 1992; Rutter 1974
Active processing of experiences	Even quite young children think about what happens to them and develop ideas about the meaning of such experiences.	There is considerable interest today in how young people view their world because this is associated with how they act on it.	Kagan 1984
Multifactorial causation	Earlier psychosocial research assumed that single risk factors were responsible for the causation of a disorder. Empirical evidence questioned this.	Fergusson and Lynskey's longitudinal studies, for example, show that increased rates of risk factors Produce up to a 100% increase in risk of an antisocial disorder.	Fergusson and Lynskey 1996

Table 1.1 – *continued*

Some key influences	Implications	Current view	Some key studies
1980s and early 1990s – *continued*			
The challenge from behavioural genetics	Differences between children in a family were mainly genetic rather than environmental. Genetic factors influenced the extent to which some children were exposed to psychosocial risk. Genetics influence liability to psychological problems, especially over time.	Although the evidence supporting the power of genetic influences has strengthened, the same evidence has shown that environmental factors play an important role. Geneticists are now more interested in the gene–environment associations.	Plomin and Daniels 1987; Scarr 1992; Plomin and Bergeman 1991; Kendler *et al.* 1993; Rutter *et al.* 1999 a,b
Resilience	There is huge individual variation in responses to stress and adversity.	Much is known about psychosocial risk factors. We have still a long way to go before we can adequately understand risk and protective processes in resilience.	Rutter in press a,b

Source: based on Rutter 1999a.

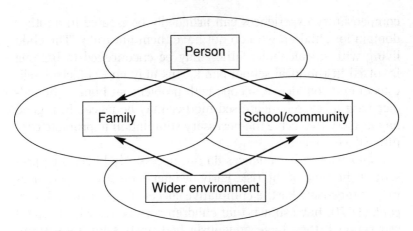

Fig. 1.3 The interacting 'ecological framework'.

rate the new ideas. Under this model the child is viewed across four domains. In each of the domains – the biological child, the family, the school/community and the wider world – known risk and protective factors for a child's emotional well-being can be identified.

Risk and protective factors are not absolute or static. In each domain they interact with each other. On the whole single stressful experiences that occur in isolation are less damaging than cumulative stresses (Rutter 1979; Emery 1982; Kolvin *et al.* 1990).

At particular moments in time a child may be developmentally more protected or developmentally more vulnerable to adversities (Rutter 1995). The cumulative effect of risk factors may be greatest where they set off a chain reaction. For example, a child with behaviour problems before entering school goes into school poorly prepared, achieves less in school, is disruptive, is suspended, and has as a result a poorer education, fewer qualifications, is less able to obtain work, becomes unemployed, is more likely be depressed in adult life. Individuals may have biological personal traits that make them more or less likely to respond positively or negatively to personal stresses. For one child a school examination may seem like a challenge to be overcome; for another the anxiety may be associated with acute distress.

The strength of thinking about children 'ecologically' is that compensatory experiences can artificially be created in another domain for children who do not have them naturally. The child living with an alcoholic father may be encouraged to become involved in the local school band. This may give sufficient self-esteem and confidence to cope with problems at home. The toddler with a severely depressed mother may be placed in a good day nursery to receive the necessary stimulation to promote cognitive development.

Compensatory experiences do not necessarily have to be present at the time of the risk. Early or later protective experiences may compensate for the cumulative effects of risk factors. Stacey *et al.* (1970) have shown that children cope better with hospital separation if they have previously had unstressful 'separation' experiences. Quinton *et al*'s (1984) study of institutionally reared children found that in later life partnership relationships could be compensatory for the early adverse experiences.

An early life free from life's adversities may in itself be a risk factor, because the young person may never develop the necessary coping mechanisms and confidence to deal with later life stresses (Seligman 1975; Hennessy and Levine 1979). Children who have never failed an examination may crumble at their first setback. Linked into this idea is that risk and protective factors have to be seen in the context of how the person cognitively processes the experiences. Two children in the same family may 'process' the experience of their parents' divorce very differently and as a result respond differently. One child may be able to cope because he accepts the 'reason' for the break-up while another may be angry because he feels rejected by the departing parent.

Specific risk and protective factors for emotional well-being

Table 1.2 lists some identified risk and protective factors for emotional and behavioural disorders.

Is resilience the X factor?

A central finding in all the literature on psychosocial adversities is that some children, despite prolonged and severely negative

Table 1.2 Some risk and protective factors for emotional and behavioural disorders

Factors in the person	Factors in the family	Factors at school/ or in the community	Wider world factors
Risk Biological factors making the children more vulnerable to problems; e.g. inherited mental illness. Temperament. Impulsiveness. Physical illness or disability. Mental disabilities. Negative attitudes to school etc.	*Risk* Family adversities: poverty; maltreatment; domestic violence; mental illness in parents; alcoholism; criminality. Conflict with, and between, parents. Lax, inconsistent supervision. Punitive, authoritarian/ inflexible parenting.	*Risk* Poor reading/low school attainment; poor rates of achievement in schools. Bullying in schools. Disadvantaged community/ neighbourhood crime/ poverty. Racial tension/ harassment. An experience of public 'care'.	*Risk* Economic recession. Unemployment. Housing shortage. Family change: increasing family breakdown; long working hours/job insecurity.
Protective Biological resilience: good health and development. Good problem-solving skills/high IQ. Planning ability: internal working models/adult attachment. Turning point decisions; i.e. to leave high risk community, gain further qualifications. Positive attitudes.	*Protective* Good relationships with parents. Supportive grandparents. Lack of domestic tensions. Family involvement in activities; 'family togetherness'. Father involvement. Being brought up in a birth family. Positive parenting.	*Protective* Supportive community. Schools with good rates of achievement; good 'ethos': lack of bullying. Opportunities for involvement and achievement.	*Protective* 'Inclusive' government policies.

Source: Buchanan and Ten Brinke 1998.

experiences, survive intact. What is this 'X' factor? What can be done to promote resilience? In promoting children's well-being promoting resilience to life's adversities is key. Recent research has taken some of the mystery out of resilience. Certainly personal attributes play a part ('the born survivor') but there is also much that can be done to improve resilience. Compas (1995), in studies on children's coping strategies, has found that one of the biggest threats to children's mental health is the *persistent* presence of minor irritants rather than occasional major stressors.

In New Zealand, the Christchurch longitudinal study compared two groups who scored highly on a family adversity index. Assessed at age 15–16, *the resilient group* had low self-reported offending ratings, police contact, conduct problems, alcohol abuse, and school drop-out, whereas *the non-resilient group* had high ratings on these factors. The first finding was that the resilient young people *had significantly lower adversity scores*. Those with multiple problems usually had the highest scores. Resilient young people tended to have higher IQs at 8 years; had lower rates of novelty seeking at age 16 and were less likely to belong to delinquent peer groups. Girls were no more resilient than boys. There was little difference between the two groups on parental attachment, and other individual features were not linked to the variations in resilience (Fergusson and Lynskey 1996).

What are the implications of this study and the findings from Compas? Firstly, even with children who experience multiple adversities, lightening the load may free up energy that can be used productively. Secondly, in adolescence the key influence is not so much the family but the peer group. Strategies to divert young people away from delinquent peer groups seem to be supported by research.

Rutter *et al.* (1998), in reviewing all the research, hypothesise that resilience in young people may be promoted by:

- *reducing sensitivity to risk* by giving young people opportunities to succeed in challenging *activities;*
- *reducing the impact of the risk* by parental supervision; positive peer-group experience; avoidance of being drawn into parental conflict; and opportunities to distance oneself from the deviant parent;

- *reducing negative chain effects* resulting, for example, from suspension from school; truancy; drug and alcohol abuse;
- *increasing positive chain effects* by eliciting supportive responses from other people; e.g. linking a young person with someone who may help in getting a job;
- *promoting self-esteem and self-efficacy* by giving young people opportunities to succeed in tasks and success in coping with manageable stresses;
- *compensatory experiences* that directly counter the risk effects; e.g. where a child has witnessed domestic violence, positive models of non-violent men;
- *opening up of positive opportunities* for example through education and career opportunities;
- *positive cognitive processing of negative experiences;* for example, teaching coping strategies and skills, viewing negative experiences positively, being constructive.

Children in the public care

A particularly vulnerable group of young people appear to be those who enter public care. In the UK and the US, the rediscovery of child abuse by Henry Kempe *et al.* (1962) brought with it an increase in the number of children who were admitted to public care. Such were the concerns about children's safety, that children were 'rescued' into the safety of children's homes and substitute parents. By the end of the 1970s some 100 000 children were being looked after by the state, around 8 in every 1000 children in the UK (Utting 1991).

In recent years in the UK, there has been a major re-evaluation. Substantial evidence has been forthcoming that the children were disadvantaged before ever they entered care, but they may have been further disadvantaged by the public parent. Cheung and Buchanan (1997), using data from the longitudinal National Child Development Study in the UK, which has data on 17 000 children born in one week in 1958, found that children who had ever been in public care had much higher rates of maladjustment at 16 than a comparative group of children brought up in severe disadvantage. Similarly in another study, Buchanan and Ten Brinke (1997) found one in five children who had been in care had a tendency to depression at age 33.

Studies by Barnardo's (1996), show that children who were being 'looked after' by the state were over-represented amongst the unemployed (50–80% of care leavers were unemployed); the underachieving (5% of care leavers had no academic qualifications); offending (23% of adult prisoners and 38% of young prisoners had been in care); teen parents (one in seven young women leaving care were pregnant or already mothers); homeless (30% of young single homeless had been in care).

The 'prevention' movement

As researchers in the US and UK increasingly demonstrated that levels of disturbance differed between groups and between schools, as well as between communities, it was hypothesised that if the risk factors could be reduced and protection increased, some problems could be prevented.

The situation in the US

Hawkins notes:

As the costs of crime, teen pregnancies, an undereducated underclass living in poverty, and substance abuse have increased, policy-makers and researchers have looked more seriously at prevention as a potentially cost-effective approach to reduce the prevalence of these behaviors. Efforts to improve schools, reduce crime and violence, combat substance abuse, and prevent unwanted pregnancies have progressed on separate tracks. (1999a, p. 226)

During the 1980s and early 1990s in the US, building on the earlier work of centres such as the Oregon Social Learning Center, groups came together; for example, The Society for Prevention Research, incorporating 'scientists, practitioners, advocates, administrators and policy makers' from all over the US who were concerned with problems, issues and challenges pertaining to the prevention of public health and social problems such as drug and alcohol abuse, psychiatric disorders, other mental problems, delinquency, crime and violence, child abuse, etc. At the same time, also in the US, the National Institute of Mental Health (NIMH) and the National Institute on Drug Abuse (NIDA) were also supporting prevention research.

These bodies have had an important role in sponsoring research at centres such as The Oregon Social Learning Center in Eugene and The Prevention Research Center at Washington University in Seattle. Hawkins in Seattle believes that:

The promotion of positive youth and adult development and the prevention of health and mental health and other problems before they emerge is really becoming a possibility in our society at this point in history. I think prevention is going to become much more central in social welfare and social work in the next ten years than it has been in the last thirty. (1999b. Internet mission statement.)

The Center proposes a five-phase model of prevention research (Fig. 1.4):

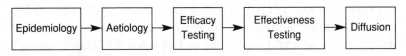

Fig. 1.4 The prevention model.

The first two phases are descriptive studies. *Epidemiology* identifies the problem or disorder and studies its distribution and prevalence in a given population. *Aetiology* identifies risk and protective factors that serve as predictors for the problem. *Efficacy Testing* involves controlled trials designed to reduce risk factors or enhance protective factors. *Effectiveness Testing* involves field trials to determine whether the intervention has the desired effects in a real-world context. The final stage, *Diffusion*, takes the proven intervention into multiple settings. In the US, for example, the Blueprint Programmes for Violence Prevention play a role in diffusion. Elliott, the series editor, reminds us:

To date most of the resources committed to the prevention and control of youth violence at both the national and local levels, has been invested in untested programs based on questionable assumptions and delivered with little consistency or quality control. Further, the vast majority of these programs are not being evaluated. This means we will never know which (if any) of them have had some significant deterrent effect; we will learn nothing from our investment in these programs to improve our understanding of the causes of violence or to guide our future efforts to deter violence; and there will be no real accountability for the expenditures of scarce community resources. Worse yet, some of the most popular programs have been demonstrated in careful scientific studies to be ineffective, and yet we continue to invest huge sums of money in them for largely political reasons. (Elliott 1998, p. xi)

The situation in the UK

In the UK, there has been a similar movement towards prevention and prevention research. At the end of the 1980s, central to this movement was the enactment of the Children Act 1989 in England and Wales. This Act, using research evidence, outlined the principles of how children should be treated under the law and under the publicly provided social services for children and families. These principles were intended to be preventive in nature.

Under Section 17(10), a child in England and Wales with emotional and behavioural problems was included under the definition of a 'child in need' and entitled to family support services. Local authorities had a duty to identify children who were 'in need' in their area.

Since the Children Act 1989, the Department of Health has invested considerable resources to discover how public services were responding to the Act. These, largely descriptive, studies demonstrated that children's services have found it difficult to move from a child protection role to a more proactive preventive role in promoting children's well-being (Department of Health 1995).

The arrival of New Labour in 1997 brought a new urgency to preventive work. At the centre of their concerns are the numbers of children and young people who for one reason or another are 'socially excluded'.

Overall, the government's approach amounts to a major public health campaign to combat the risk factors for psychological disturbance and to promote the protective resources associated with emotional well-being in children.

The government is committed to ending child poverty, tackling social exclusion and promoting the welfare of all children so that they can thrive and fulfil their potential as citizens throughout their lives.

Programmes such as Sure Start and Quality Protects and policies to support families, promote educational attainment, cut truancy and school exclusion and secure a future for young people not in education, employment or training all aim to ensure that children and families most at risk of social exclusion have every opportunity to build successful, independent lives . . .

Promoting the well-being of children to ensure their optimal outcomes requires integration at both national and local levels: joined up government – in respect both of policy making and of service delivery – is central to the current extensive policy agenda. (Department of Health 1999)

Effectively these huge cross-departmental programmes – 'joined up solutions to joined up problems' – are designed to promote the well-being of communities who in the past may have not done so well. At the centre of all programmes are projects to support parents and to improve their skills.

Comparing the situation in the US with that in the UK

Whereas in the US there is now a body of preventive research showing what works, from the perspective of the five-stage prevention research model the UK is largely still at stages one and two – descriptive studies.

Thanks largely to our longitudinal national birth cohort studies, such as The National Child Development Study, we are quite well informed about the *epidemiology* and *aetiology of* our social problems. The government has also invested in a number of descriptive studies showing how our national and local services are responding to the problems (e.g. Department of Health 1995). There have, however, been remarkably few randomised controlled trials.

In the UK, however, we are in the happy position of having a government prepared to invest significant resources in national programmes to promote children's emotional well-being and to combat 'social exclusion'. The concern is that resources are being spent on major initiatives, such as *Sure Start* and *On Target* – a programme to prevent crime by supporting families and children – without having undertaken the necessary stage three of preventive research: *efficacy testing*.

Many of these government programmes are based on programmes from the US. Since, on a number of indicators, such as violent crime, substance abuse and teen pregnancies, rates in the UK are still below those in the US, there may be specific factors in the UK that explain these. We do not know how well the carefully validated US programmes cross the cultural gap. The danger is that without UK studies unproven and possibly even harmful interventions in children's lives will be allowed to take place. The related concern is that if the current initiatives being undertaken by the UK government fail to deliver, it may be a long time before another opportunity presents to promote children's emotional and behavioural well-being.

The outline of this book

This book highlights recent and current research being undertaken in the UK to remedy this gap in research. The book reflects the interdisciplinary movement seen in prevention research in the US and the 'joined up' philosophy of the current UK government.

The following chapters are written or co-authored by leading researchers in their fields. In most chapters there is both a summary of past research by others working in their area, and an outline of their current work. In Chapter 2, Sarah Stewart-Brown takes a public health perspective emphasising the importance of well-being to society as a whole. The next chapter summarises studies relating to the prevalence of children with emotional and behavioural disorders and then uses data from the National Child Development Study to make two points: firstly large numbers of children have emotional and behavioural problems while growing up but many 'recover'. The challenge for interventions, therefore, is to improve on this natural 'recovery' rate. In Chapter 4, Adrienne Katz's 'Promoting our well-being: young views' gives a very strong message through the perspectives of young people. The following two chapters move into parenting research. Frances Gardner and Sarah Ward outline research on conduct disorders, particularly that relating to Patterson's 'coercive theory'. The Gardner–Ward chapter breaks new ground in exploring how to help children develop the values and skills necessary to promote their own and others' future well-being. Roger Grimshaw highlights the key principles in implementing effective parenting programmes. In the next chapter Catherine Baillie, Kathy Sylva and Emma Evans make the link between home and school in describing a new programme to improve children's reading skills while helping parents manage their children's behaviour. Jane Wells moves us right into the school with a systematic review of studies to improve emotional well-being in schools. Joan Hunt takes us further along our journey, reminding us that when parenting breaks down, the state, as the public parent, intervenes. Although the court, under the Children Act 1989 in England and Wales, is mandated to safeguard and promote the child's welfare, the socio-legal system can have unintended consequences. Finally Deborah Capaldi and Mark Eddy look back over thirty years of research at the Oregon Social Learning Center, the place where so many of the ideas now promoted in this book originated. They take us on a journey into the future, looking at the continuities and discontinuities of adolescence and adult life, and they share with us the findings from their latest research highlighting new directions in their interventions. The many messages from the research on ways to promote the well-being of this and future generations of children and young people are summarised in the last chapter.

References

Albee, G. (1992). Saving Children means social revolutions. In G. W. Albee, L. Bond and T. C. Monsey (eds.), *Improving children's lives: global perspectives on prevention*, p. 327. Newbury, PRK, Sage.

Baldwin, A. L. (1968). *Theories of child development*. New York, Wiley.

Bandura, A. and Walters, R. H. (1963). *Social learning and personality development*. New York, Rinehart and Winston.

Barker, R. G. and Wright, H. F. (1955). *The Midwest and its children*. New York, Harper and Row.

Barnardo's (1996). *Too much – too young; the failure of social policy in meeting the needs of care leavers*. Action on Aftercare Consortium, London, Barnardo's.

Bowlby, J. (1951). *Maternal care and mental health*. Geneva, WHO.

Bronfenbrenner, U. (1979). *The ecology of human development: Experiments in nature and design*. Cambridge, MA. Harvard University Press.

Brown, G. W. and Harris, T. O. (1978). *Social origins of depression: A study of psychiatric disorder in women.* London, Tavistock.

Buchanan, A. (1996). *Cycles of child maltreatment: facts, fallacies and interventions.* Chichester, Wiley.

Buchanan, A. (1999). *What works for troubled children: family support for children with emotional and behavioural problems.* London, Barnardo's.

Buchanan, A. and Hudson, B. L. (eds.) (1998). *Parenting, schooling and children's behaviour,* Aldershot, Ashgate.

Buchanan, A. and Ten Brinke, J-A. (1997). *What happened when they were grown up? Outcomes from parenting experiences.* York, Joseph Rowntree Foundation/York Publishing.

Buchanan, A. and Ten Brinke, J-A. (1998). *'Recovery' from emotional and behavioural problems.* Report to NHS Executive Anglia and Oxford.

Cabinet Office (1998). *Truancy and school exclusion.* Report by the Social Exclusion Unit. London, HMSO.

Cheung, S. Y. and Buchanan, A. (1997). Malaise scores in adulthood of children and young people who have been in care. *Journal of Child Psychology and Psychiatry,* **38**(5), 575–80.

Children Act 1989. London, HMSO.

Clarke, A. M. and Clarke, A. D. B. (1976). *Early experience: myths and evidence.* London, Open Books.

Compas, B. E. (1995). Promoting successful coping during adolescence. In M. Rutter (ed.), *Psychosocial disturbances in young people,* Cambridge, Press Syndicate of University of Cambridge, pp. 247–73.

Conger, R. D., Conger, K. J., Elder, G. H., *et al.* (1992). A family process model of economic hardship and adjustment of early adolescent boys. *Child Development,* **63**(3), 526–41.

Dare, C. (1976). Psychoanalytic theories. In M. Rutter and L. Hersov (eds.), *Child psychiatry: modern approaches,* pp. 255–68. Oxford, Blackwell Scientific.

Department of Education and Employment (1999). *Blunkett congratulates GCSE and Part One GNVQ Students,* Press Release 389/99. 29 August. HMSO.

Department of Health (1995). *Child protection: Messages from research.* London. The Stationery Office.

Department of Health (1999). *A framework for the assessment of children in need and their families: a consultation draft.*

Elliott, D. S. (series ed.) (1998). *Blueprints for violence prevention,* Venture, Gold, CO.

Emery, R. E. (1982). Interparental conflict and the child of discord and divorce. *Psychological Bulletin,* **92**, 310–30.

Farrington, D. (1988). Studying changes within individuals: the causes of offending. In M. Rutter (ed.), *Studies of psychosocial risk: the power of longitudinal data,* pp. 158–83. Cambridge, Cambridge University Press.

Fergusson, D. M. and Lynskey, M. T. (1996). Adolescent resilience to family adversity. *Journal of Child Psychology and Psychiatry*, **9**(4), 483–94.

Freud, A. and Dann, S. (1951). An experiment in group upbringing. *Psychoanalytical Study of the Child*, **6**, 127–68.

Gullotta, T. P., Hampton, R. L. Sentore, V. and Eissmann, M. (1999). When Pap get too handy with his Hick'ry. In R. L. Hampton, V. Sentore, T. P. Gullotta, *Substance abuse, family violence and child welfare*. California Park, Sage.

Harlow, H. F. (1958). The nature of love. *American Psychologist*, **13**, 673–85.

Hawkins, D. (1999a). Preventing adolescent health-risk behaviors by strengthening protection during childhood. *Archives of Pediatrics and Adolescent Medicine*, **153**, 222–34.

Hawkins, D. (1999b). Mission Statement. Center for Prevention Research. *Weber.u.washington.edu. swprc*.

Hennessy, J. W. and Levine, S. (1979). Stress, arousal, and the pituitary-adrenal system: a psycho-endocrine hypothesis. In J. M. Srague and S. A. N. Epstein (eds.), *Progress in psychobiology and physiological psychology*, pp. 134–78. New York, Academic.

Hewitt, L. and Jenkins, R. L. (1946). *Fundamental patterns of maladjustment*. Illinois, Michigan Child Guidance Institute.

Home Office (1998). *Supporting families*. London, Home Office.

Illich, I. (1973). *Deschooling society*. Harmondsworth, Penguin.

Kagan, J. (1984; rep. 1994). *The nature of the child*. New York, Basic.

Kempe, C. H., Silverman, F., Steele, B., *et al.* (1962). The battered child syndrome. *Journal of the American Medical Association*, **181**, 17–24.

Kendler, K. S., Kessler, R. C., Neale, M. C., *et al.* (1993). The prediction of major depression in women: toward an integrated etiologic model. *American Journal of Psychiatry*, **150**(8), 1139–48.

Kolvin, I., Miller, F. J. W., Scott, D. M., *et al.* (1990). *Continuities of deprivation? The Newcastle 1000 family study*. Aldershot, Avebury.

Kovacs, M. and Devlin, B. (1998). Internalizing disorders in childhood. *Journal of Child Psychology and Psychiatry*, **39**(1), 47–63.

Leahy, A. M. (1935). Nature-nurture and intelligence. *Genetic Psychology Monographs*. **17**, 236–308.

Levine, S. (1962). The effects of infantile experience on adult behavior. In A. J. Bachrach (ed.), *Experimental foundations of clinical psychology*. New York, Basic.

Loeber, R. and LeBlanc, M. (1990). Towards a developmental criminology. In M. Tonry and N. Morris (eds.), *Crime and Justice*, pp. 375–473. Chicago, University of Chicago Press.

Macintyre, S. and Ellaway, A. (1999). Ecological approaches. Rediscovering the role of the physical and social environment. In L. Berkman and I. Kawachi (eds.), *Social epidemiology*, Chapt. 14. Oxford, Oxford University Press.

Maughan, B. (1994). School influences. In M. Rutter and D. F. Hay (eds.), *Development through life: a handbook for clinicians*, pp. 134–58. Oxford, Blackwell Scientific.

Miller, N. E. and Dollard, J. (1941). *Social learning and imitation*. New York, McGraw-Hill.

Mortimore, P. P. (1995). The positive influence of schooling. In M. Rutter (ed), *Psychosocial disturbance in young people: challenges for prevention*, pp. 333–63. New York, Cambridge University Press.

Plomin, R., and Bergeman, C. S. (1991). The nature of nurture: genetic influence on 'environmental' measures. *Behavioral and Brain Sciences*, **14**, 3373–427.

Plomin, R. and Daniels, D. (1987). Why are children in the same family so different from one another? *Behavioral and Brain Sciences*, **10**, 1–16.

Quinton, D., Rutter, M. and Liddle, C. (1984). Institutional rearing, parenting difficulties and marital support. *Psychological Medicine*, **14**, 107–24.

Robins, L. N. (1986). Changes in conduct disorder over time. In D. C. Farran and J. D. McKinney (eds.), *Risk and intellectual and social development*, pp. 227–59. New York, Academic.

Rowe, D. C. (1994). *The limits of family influence: genes, experience and behavior*. New York, Guildford.

Rutter, M. (1974). Dimensions of parenthood: some myths and some suggestions. In *The family in society*. Department of Health and Social Security, London, HMSO.

Rutter, M. (1979). Protective factors in children's responses to stress and disadvantages. In M. W. Kent and E. Rolf (eds.), *Primary prevention of psychopathology III: social competence in children*, pp. 49–74. Hanover, NH, University Press of New England.

Rutter, M. (1995). Causal concepts and their testing. In M. Rutter and D. Smith (eds.), *Psychosocial disorders in young people: time trends and their causes*, pp. 7–34. Chichester, Wiley.

Rutter, M. (1999a). Psychosocial adversity and child psychopathology. *British Journal of Psychiatry*, **174**, 480–93.

Rutter, M. (1999b). Resilience reconsidered: conceptual considerations and empirical findings. In J. P. Shonkoff and A. S. Meisels (eds.), *Handbook of early childhood interventions*. 2nd edn. New York, Cambridge University Press.

Rutter, M. and Quinton, D. (1977). Psychiatric disorder – ecological factors and concepts of causation. In H. McGurk (ed.), *Ecological factors in human development*, pp. 173–87. Amsterdam, North-Holland.

Rutter, M. and Smith, D. (1995). *Psychosocial disorders in young people: time, trends and their causes*, Chichester, Wiley.

Rutter, M., Tizard, B. and Whitmore, K. (1970). *Education, health and behaviour*, London, Longman.

Rutter, M., Maughan, B. and Mortimore, P. (1979). *Fifteen thousand hours: secondary schools and their effects on children*. Cambridge, MA. Harvard University Press.

Rutter, M., Giller, H. and Hagell, A. (1998). *Antisocial behaviour by young people.* University of Cambridge Press.

Rutter, M., Silberg, R. J., O'Connor, T., *et al.* (1999). Genetics and child psychiatry: I empirical research findings. *Journal of Child Psychology and Psychiatry Review,* **40**, 19–55.

Scarr, S. (1992). Developmental theories for the 1990s development and individual differences. *Child Development,* **63**, 1–19.

Scarr, S. (1997) Behavior-genetic and socialization theories of intelligence: truth and reconciliation. In R. J. Sternberg and E. L. Grigorenko (eds.), *Intelligence, heredity and environment,* pp. 3–41. Cambridge, Cambridge University Press.

Seligman, M. (1975). *Helplessness: on depression, development and death.* San Francisco, Freeman.

Simeonsson, R. (1994). Promoting health, education and well-being. In R. Simeonsson (ed.), *Risk, resilience and prevention: promotion of the well-being of children.* Baltimore, Brookes.

Skeels, H. M. and Dye, H. (1939). A study of the effects of differential stimulation on mentally retarded children. *Proceedings of the American Association of Mental Deficiency,* **44**, 114–36.

Skinner, B. F. (1938). *The behavior of organisms: on experimental analysis.* New York, Appleton-Century-Crofts.

Spivack, G., Marcus, J. and Swift, M. (1986). Early classroom behaviors and later misconduct. *Developmental Psychology,* **22**, 124–31.

Stacey, M., Dearden, R., Pill, R. and Robinson, D. (1970). *Hospital, children and their families. The report of a pilot study.* London, Routledge.

Stainton Rogers, R. (1989). The social construction of childhood. In W. Stainton Rogers, D. Hevy and E. Ash (eds.), *Child abuse and neglect,* pp 23–9. Batsford, Open University,

Thomas, E. A. C., Chess, S., and Birch, H. G. (1968). *Temperament and behavior disorders in childhood.* New York, New York University Press.

Tizard, J., Sinclair, I. and Clarke, R. V. G. (eds.) (1975). *Varieties of residential experience.* London, Routledge and Kegan Paul.

Tremblay, R. E., LeBlanc, M., and Schwartzman, A. E. (1988). The predictive power of the first-grade peer and teacher ratings of behavior: sex differences in antisocial behavior and personality at adolescence. *Journal of Abnormal Child Psychology,* **16**, 571–83.

U.N. General Assembly. (1989). *Adoption of a Convention on the rights of the child.* (U.N. Doc. A/Res. 44/45). New York, United Nations.

Utting, W. (1991). *Children in the public care.* London, HMSO.

Van Ijzendoorn, M. H. (1995). Adult attachment representations, parental responsiveness, and infant attachment: a meta-analysis on the predictive validity of the Adult Attachment Interview. *Psychological Bulletin,* **116**, 387–403.

Wootton, B. (1959). *Social science and social pathology.* London, Allen and Unwin.

2

Parenting, well-being, health and disease

Sarah Stewart-Brown

'Parenting is probably the most important public health issue facing our society.' Hoghughi 1998

Parenting, well-being, health and disease are all concepts in common household use: 'I am taking care of the children this afternoon', 'I don't feel well today', 'My health is important to me', 'I have a disease called . . .'. Yet the task of defining each of these four has been the subject of many books, theses, and academic papers. The aim of this chapter – to develop a model, suggesting that all four are inextricably linked – is therefore a bold one, particularly as it will not be possible in the space available to review all that has been written about each concept.

The chapter will offer working definitions of all four concepts, explain the model which links the four together, describe some of the increasing number of studies which support the centrality of parenting in the model, and suggest ways in which future studies might test the model further. It will provide evidence to suggest that the promotion of children's emotional well-being is important for improving public health as well as for reducing violence and criminality, child abuse and academic failure. There is a growing literature on the role that teachers and teaching play in the development of emotional well-being in childhood (see Chapter 8, and Weare 2000), and the model presented in this chapter could be expanded to include schools and teachers. There is also a large literature demonstrating the importance of the physical and cognitive aspects of parenting – feeding, safety, conversation and play – in child development. Because of constraints on space this chapter will not cover either of these, concentrating on the role of parents and parenting in emotional rather than physical or intellectual development.

Definitions

Health and disease

The three principal models of health are described by Mildred Blaxter in her book *Health and lifestyles* (1990). The first is implicit in the beliefs and writings of the medical profession: that health is the absence of disease. In this model, health is something people have when they do not have an illness or disease. A doctor's diagnosis is an important part of the definition of illness or disease, and the identification of biomedical causes an important part of diagnosis. There are a number of problems in applying this definition in practice because people with no disease may feel unwell, and people who have diseases such as early cancers, epilepsy or hypertension may feel well.

The second definition is based on functionality or ability to cope. The concepts of resilience, reserves and resources are important in this model, which focuses on what people can or cannot do, rather than on what doctors consider to be wrong with them. This is the model adopted by those working in the discipline of health promotion in the Ottawa Charter (WHO 1986).

The third definition is that proposed by the WHO in the late 1940s (1947). In this, health is defined as a state of complete physical, mental and social well-being, not merely the absence of disease. The presence or absence of health is determined by the subjective assessment of the individual concerned, not by the objective assessment of others. One problem with the WHO definition of health is that it appears to define a state which is not common. There are therefore concerns about its attainability, and about the responsibility of the government towards its citizens in this respect. The policies of the NHS and the practice

of health professionals suggest that the latter may attribute
greater legitimacy and value to the attainment of physical well-
being – stamina, flexibility, strength and freedom from pain –
than to the attainment of social or mental well-being. It is
implicit in the model which this chapter describes, that all three
are essential to health.

Well-being

In one way well-being is a simple concept. A moment's reflection
provides an answer to the question 'Do I feel well?' The answers
appear to range from 'No, I feel (at varying levels of severity)
tired/irritable/anxious/low/in pain, etc.' to 'Yes, I feel well'. In
other ways, as evidenced by the extensive, wide-ranging and diffuse academic literature (see Andrews and Robinson 1991), the
concept is clearly complex, covering a number of other concepts
including quality of life, life satisfaction, happiness and morale.
In the academic tradition, this literature is primarily devoted to
developing methods of defining and measuring well-being in
others, rather than subjective reflection on what well-being feels
like. If well-being is more easily understood through subjective
reflection than through observation of others, it is perhaps not
surprising that the academic approach has proved difficult.

   Mental and social well-being are arguably more diffuse concepts than physical well-being and their relationship to mental
illness, to mental and psychological health and to emotional
well-being needs to be clarified (see Weare 2000 and Tudor
1996 for a fuller discussion). Whilst it is used by some as an
overarching concept, covering emotional and social well-being,
the term 'mental health' causes problems because it has been
used to describe the NHS services for the mentally ill and does
not have much public credence (Pavis *et al.* 1996). Mental illness
is defined in terms of objectively quantifiable criteria based on
doctors' observations of patients' behaviour, and their reported
thoughts and feelings (American Psychiatric Association, DSM
IV 1987). Mental well-being has two components: cognitive
(thinking clearly, logically and creatively) and affective (feeling,
for example, happy, calm, energetic). Both of these are primarily
subjective states, but the effect of their absence can be observed

objectively in people's behaviour and communication. Psychological health also seems to combine both objective and subjective aspects; some psychologists use objective observation of behaviour to measure health, while others develop standardised measures of how people feel. Emotional well-being, on the other hand, is concerned only with feelings and is therefore essentially subjective.

There is a growing academic literature that attempts to define and describe aspects of social well-being and to measure their impact on health and disease. One aspect – social capital – describes communities which demonstrate norms of participation, equality and social trust (Bruhn and Rolfs 1979; Putnam *et al.* 1993), places where people look out for one another and expect to both give and receive help and support when needed. Another aspect – social support (Berkman and Syme 1979; Seeman and Syme 1987; Cohen 1988; Berkman 1995) – describes the number and quality of relationships between people in families and communities. Both of these can be shown to have an impact on the incidence of, and mortality from, a range of common and important health problems and diseases (see Wilkinson 1996, for further reading).

A definition of social well-being which covers all these approaches, and is the one used in the model developed in this chapter, is 'relationships between people which enhance, rather than damage, the well-being of individuals'. Practitioners and academics in the discipline of psychotherapy have suggested on the basis of clinical experience and observational research that effective therapeutic relationships are those which are built on the respect, empathy and genuineness of the therapist towards the client (Rogers 1959; Egan 1982; Davis 1993). It is not too great a step to suggest that relationships which enhance, rather than damage, individual well-being are likely to be those which are mutually respectful, empathetic and genuine. Family violence, drug and alcohol misuse, theft, fraud, mugging, vandalism, dishonesty, lack of respect and lack of compassion are therefore all aspects of social 'disease'.

There is a growing body of research which suggests that emotional literacy (which enables the development of emotional intelligence) (Steiner 1997) is a key skill in the development of interpersonal relationships (Goleman 1996; Stone *et al.* 1999), in the maintenance of health (Goleman 1996; Ornish 1998), and in the creation of effective workplaces (Goleman 1998) and schools (Weare 2000). Emotional literacy is made up of three abilities: the ability to understand personal emotions, the ability to listen to others and to empathise with their emotions, and the ability to express emotions productively (Steiner 1997).

In this chapter the term well-being is used to describe a holistic, subjective state which is present when a range of feelings, among them energy, confidence, openness, enjoyment, happiness, calm and caring, are combined and balanced. People who feel like this are likely to relate to other people in a way that enhances their own and other people's health.

Parenting

Parenting is another term whose meaning is apparently self-evident, yet is widely debated. Much of the debate centres on the importance of different parental behaviours for child health and development. If certain behaviours can be demonstrated to have a negative impact on child health and development then it can be argued that parents have a responsibility not to behave in these ways. It is only relatively recently that the importance of parenting has been recognised to the extent that the subject attracts research investment. Prior to that, parenting practices were developed on the basis of experiential knowledge, together with pedagogic teaching. Parenting knowledge was handed down from generation to generation within communities. When research evidence conflicts with experiential knowledge or theoretical beliefs, it is likely to generate intense social debate. It is not surprising, therefore, that the subject of parenting generates debate. It is also not surprising that parents who were subjected to physical punishment as a normal part of their own childhood, who have been taught that physical punishment is the right way to discipline children, and who have observed, in their own families, that violence is an effective short-term solution, greet with disbelief research evidence suggesting that physical punishment is detrimental to children's long-term development. Adult behaviour is difficult to change, and even adults who accept such research evidence in principle may find it difficult to behave differently. The guilt engendered by recognising that a particular personal behaviour could be harmful to their children may play a role in rejection of the principle.

The best-established research base on parenting has been developed by child psychiatrists and psychologists (see below). This shows that a small number of parenting practices are associated with emotional and behavioural problems in children. There are several schools of thought about what causes this association. The first two both suggest that the problem begins with parents. The behaviourist approach is based on the belief that parents parent in unhelpful ways through ignorance, developed from mistaken teaching and from unhelpful role models (their own and other people's parents). The second, the psychotherapeutic approach, is based on the belief that parents parent in unhelpful ways because they feel distressed and unsupported. The competing school of thought believes that the problem begins with babies, suggesting that genetically determined neuro-psychological or temperamental differences between babies make parenting more or less difficult and cause unhelpful parenting practices. These different schools of thought all accept the experimental evidence that interventions which are successful in changing parental behaviours have an important impact on children's behaviour (Barlow and Stewart-Brown, in press), but have different theories about how this change is most easily achieved (Smith 1996). One group believes that the most important element of effectiveness is helping parents learn behaviour management techniques. (Utting *et al.* 1993; Webster-Stratton 1999). A cornerstone of behaviour management is that socially desirable behaviour is rewarded and socially undesirable behaviour ignored, on the principle that what you pay attention to is what you get more of.

The second group believes that it is the nature of the relationship between parent and child which is critical, and that effective parenting is emotionally literate parenting (Gordon 1975; Gottman and Declaire 1997). Parents who treat their children with respect, empathy and genuineness understand the cause of problem behaviour and respond helpfully rather than unhelpfully, enabling children to learn to express their emotions in ways which are helpful to themselves and to their relationships with others. Rewarding desirable behaviour and ignoring undesirable behaviour is one of a number of helpful responses. This approach enables parents to develop more satisfying relationships with their children and also with other adults, and ultimately to develop greater emotional well-being. There are studies which provide evidence to support both models, and both groups would agree that poor self-esteem coupled with feelings of guilt and inadequacy are important barriers to behaviour change. The research on parenting and parenting programmes is therefore producing suggestions for healthy parent–child relationships which have much in common with those suggested by researchers working on social well-being in communities and societies (Wilkinson 1996) and in schools (Weare 2000). The feelings and behaviours that determine healthy adult relationships appear to be the same as those that determine both healthy parenting and teaching. The goal of healthy parenting can be seen as the creation of social well-being in the home, and the key skill for the development of all three is emotional literacy.

For the purposes of this chapter, parenting is therefore defined as the feelings, attitudes, beliefs and behaviours of parents towards their children.

The model

The model of well-being proposed in this chapter (Fig. 2.1) has the emotional well-being of children at its heart, and suggests that this is determined primarily by the way children are treated by their parents during childhood, manifested by social well-being in homes. If children are parented with respect, empathy and genuineness, they experience emotional well-being, and develop ways of relating to others that enhance their own and others' well-being. They grow up to be people who feel well much of the time, and who have the emotional and social resources to respond to life events and to unhelpful behaviour in others, in ways which make it likely that they will remain so. Childhood emotional well-being therefore determines adult emotional well-being.

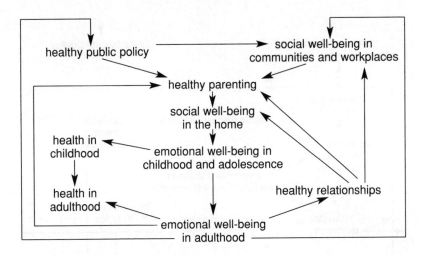

Fig. 2.1 The well-being model.

Adult emotional well-being is the primary determinant of the quality of adult relationships and therefore of social well-being in communities and societies. It also determines adults' beliefs about what motivates other people's behaviour. It thus has an important effect on the shape of public policy as determined by politicians, on management styles in workplaces, on approaches to motivation in schools, and on the level of support communities afford to parents. Parenting in the Western world is heavily constrained by social policies and norms, which are not necessarily in the interests of children or parents. These determine the social and financial support afforded to people who undertake the difficult and demanding job of parenting. They also determine the time and energy which parents can devote to caring for their children. The development of social well-being in the home by parents is therefore dependent not just on parents' emotional well-being, but also on social and workplace policies.

What happens when this goes wrong? The second model (Fig. 2.2) builds on the observation that adults who are coping with feelings of distress are more likely to behave towards others, including their children, in ways which may offer a short-term defence against distress, but are destructive and unhelpful in the longer term (that is, with lack of respect, empathy and/or genuineness).

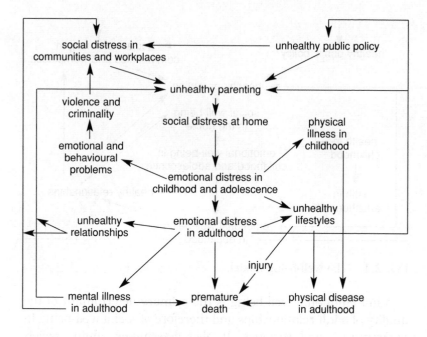

Fig. 2.2 Unhealthy societies.

The distress that this generates in other adults and children may be manifested in turn by destructive and unhelpful behaviour on their part, starting an unhelpful spiral. Feelings of distress in adults are derived in part from their perception of their relationship with others. This is influenced both by their expectations of relationships, developed in their own childhood, and by current social norms. Parents who are required by society to parent under financial, social or work-related stresses, who have either financial security or time to devote to their families, but not both, will find it more difficult to create social well-being in their homes.

Destructive and unhelpful behaviours may be self-harming or harmful to others, and are ultimately likely to be both. In childhood self-harming behaviour is manifest as 'neurotic' or 'internalising' behaviour problems. In adulthood self-harming behaviour manifests as addiction, depression, suicide attempts, anxiety, self mutilation, lack of self-care and adoption of unhealthy lifestyles. These in turn lead to disease and premature death. All these behaviours offer short-term relief from distress, but carry a significant long-term risk to health and well-being. They have a secondary impact on the well-being of others because they may be experienced as very distressing by family or friends.

Behaviour which is harmful to others is manifested in childhood by conduct disorder and Oppositional Defiance Disorder. In adulthood such behaviour is manifest by physical or emotional violence towards other people or their property, and by deceit, theft, fraud or coercion. Such behaviour also offers short-term relief from distress, but carries a serious risk to relationships. Such behaviour may be primarily damaging to other people's health and well-being in the short term; ultimately because of the way in which it damages relationships it will also impact on the distressed person's well-being and health. At present only the extremes of this behaviour – physical violence, theft and fraud – have been defined as unacceptable in law. The impact of less extreme 'personality' or 'behaviour' problems on relationships, on social well-being and on health can be demonstrated in epidemiological studies (see below). In this model, therefore, emotional distress also has an impact on physical health and well-being through the adoption of unhealthy lifestyles, through injury and also through a range of biological mechanisms such as suppression of the immune response, the development of hypertension, and possibly through interference with clotting mechanisms and musculo-skeletal tension or wear and tear (Brunner 1997).

Behaviour patterns established in childhood are difficult to change and the relationships children experience in the home are therefore critically important for the prevention of all these problems. Parents who are well supported by the communities and societies in which they live are more likely to be able to unlearn any unhelpful behavioural responses they learned in their childhood and to develop more helpful responses. Multifaceted approaches are regarded as an important component of effectiveness in health promotion (WHO 1986), and in reversing the downward spiral inherent in this model multifaceted approaches are likely to be required. The combination of interventions most likely to be effective is: personal support for parents to increase parental well-being; the development of new parenting skills, particularly emotional literacy; political policies which enable parents to have both financial security and time with their children; and social policies which support the development of social well-being in communities.

Research evidence in support of the models

As research has focussed much more strongly on health and social *problems* than on well-being, there is little research evidence to support the well-being model shown in Fig. 2.1. The justification for this model lies primarily in the experience of individuals, and of practitioners of emotional literacy and psychotherapy. There is nevertheless a growing body of research evidence to support the model that depicts what goes wrong when parents are not able to create social well-being in the home (Fig 2.2). Even in this model, however, the evidence is stronger at the periphery, where there are unequivocal problems, than it is at the centre, where the problems may be covert.

The impact of parenting on emotional and behavioural problems in childhood and on mental and social disease in adulthood

Researchers in the disciplines of child psychiatry, health psychology and criminology have created an impressive body of literature showing that certain 'parenting styles' are a cause of childhood emotional and behavioural problems. This evidence base stretches over thirty years (McCord 1963; Loeber 1983; Patterson 1989; Loeber and Dishion 1997). Structural equation models, developed from some of these studies, show that a small number of parenting practices can account for 30–40% of anti-social behaviour in children and adolescents (Patterson 1989). These same parenting styles have been shown in further models to be predictors of male violence towards female partners

(Capaldi and Clark, in press). The growing number of studies which show that it is possible to reduce emotional and behavioural problems, using interventions which aim to change parents' behaviours (Barlow and Stewart-Brown, in press) add weight to the evidence that the relationship is causal. The key attributes of parental behaviour investigated in these studies are lack of positive regard, lack of warmth, inconsistent discipline, harsh discipline, and poor monitoring and supervision.

There are also a number of studies going back a long way which show that children with emotional and behavioural problems grow up to be people who resort to criminality and violence to support themselves in adult life (Robins 1981; Stewart 1985; Farrington 1994; Loeber and Dishion 1997; Moffit *et al.* 1996). Another group has shown that aggressive and antisocial children are more likely to interpret the intentions and actions of others as hostile, that their problem-solving skills are poor, and that they have a deficient repertoire of behavioural responses (Offord and Bennett 1994). Such children have a handicap when it comes to forming positive relationships with their peers.

Evidence supporting this link between childhood behaviour problems and social and mental well-being in adulthood has also been presented from a research group who believe that antisocial behaviour in childhood is primarily attributable to genetic differences in children. This group have published studies showing that behavioural observations at age 3 years predict antisocial personality disorder and depression at age 21 (Caspi *et al.* 1996). This group have also shown in the same cohort that 'temperament' at age 3 years predicts 'personality' in young adulthood (Caspi and Silva 1995) and that 'aggressive and alienated personality' predicts violent crime, dangerous driving habits, unsafe sex, and substance misuse in 18-year-olds (Caspi *et al.* 1995).

One group of researchers has tied together these two groups of studies by documenting the progression from 'poor' parenting, through emotional and behavioural problems in early childhood, to academic failure and rejection by peers in middle childhood and to delinquency in adolescence (Patterson *et al.* 1993). More attention has been paid in this series of studies to the antecedents of antisocial behaviour in men, but there are also longitudinal follow-up studies showing that behaviour problems in childhood and adolescence predict depression in adulthood in both sexes (Bardone *et al.* 1996; Capaldi and Stoolmiller, 1999).

The impact of parenting on psychological health and health-related lifestyles in adolescence

Another group of theorists has developed a related, but different typology of parenting styles, based on discipline, nurturance, reinforcement and acceptance (Becker 1964; Dornbusch *et al.* 1987; Kelly 1983; Steinberg *et al.* 1989). Three different parenting styles have been described by this group: authoritative, permissive and authoritarian (Baumrind 1966; Baumrind 1971; Baumrind 1978; Baumrind 1991). Authoritative parenting is both responsive and restrictive, but in a way which is fair, clearly explained, consistent, and balanced to take the needs of the parents and children into account. Permissive parenting is non-restrictive, responsive and accepting; the child is effectively free from restraint. Authoritarian parenting is restrictive and demanding; conformity is valued above individuality, and discipline is often punitive. The outcome of principal interest in this research has been educational achievement, but aspects of psychological health, social competency and adolescent behaviour have also been covered. Authoritative parenting has been shown in a number of studies, both cross-sectional and longitudinal, to be associated with more robust self-concept. For example, based on responses by American children in eighth and ninth grade to a perceived parenting styles inventory, authoritative parenting has been shown to be associated with a more internal locus of control and greater self-concept on the Harter Scale (scholastic competence, social acceptance, close friendships, behavioural conduct and global self-worth), when compared to permissive or authoritarian parenting (McClun 1998). Another American research project (Cohen *et al.* 1994) has studied two independent cohorts of over 1000 children, measuring a range of independent variables and identified positive parent–child relationships (child report of praise, encouragement, physical affection, good communication and time spent with parents) in sixth and seventh graders as protective against disruptive behaviour and misuse of all substances in eighth and ninth grade. A qualitative study in the USA based on interviews with 124 adolescents and their parents also found that a high degree of parental nurturance was protective against alcohol misuse and other 'deviant' behaviours (Barnes 1984). There is a large body of literature, well accepted by practitioners and academics, that addiction to substances such as alcohol, cigarettes and drugs during adolescence increases long-term risk of physical health problems.

The impact of parenting on physical health in adulthood

The belief that the quality of human relationships, developed from learned responses in childhood, might be a risk factor for physical disease in adulthood goes back a long way (LeShan 1966). A number of other retrospective studies since that time have confirmed the relationship. More recently two prospective, longitudinal studies have been published in which measures of subjects' relationship with their parents were collected in late adolescence, and data on physical diseases was gathered subsequently. The first was a follow-up of over 1000 male medical students at Johns Hopkins University, which began in the 1950s. Their responses to a family attitude questionnaire and closeness to parents scale predicted the development of cancer in middle age. The predictive power was stronger for the more life-threatening cancers, and remained after adjustment for other cancer risk factors such as smoking and radiation exposure (Graves 1991). The second study was based on 100 male students at Harvard University. In this study three independent measures of the quality of 'parental caring', collected whilst the men were at Harvard in the 1950s, predicted doctor-diagnosed illness 35 years later. The risk was increased three to fourfold and was shown to be independent of family history of illness, smoking and the subject's marital history. The authors demonstrated a dose–response relationship of parental caring with physical health in middle age (Russek and Schwartz 1997a, b). A further longitudinal study has shown that family dissension during childhood predicts illness in later life. The odds ratios for illnesses predicted by 'dissension' were greater than those for indicators of socio-economic deprivation such as family size, broken family or economic hardship and the predictive power of dissension remained after these indicators of socio-economic deprivation have been taken into account (Lundberg 1993). There are, in addition, a number of intervention studies which add to the body of evidence suggesting that parenting could have an impact on physical health in adulthood. By demonstrating that the provision of support for parents can reduce injury rates and improve diet, they confirm the aetiological role of some aspects of parenting in the development of risk factors for subsequent physical disease or disability (Ciliska *et al.* 1994; Roberts *et al.* 1996).

Testing the model: future research

The research evidence to support the well-being model, proposed in this chapter, is most convincing in demonstrating the impact that parenting can have on the development of violence and criminality and thus on social well-being. In this area there are research studies which fulfil all the epidemiological criteria for demonstrating causality.[1] The evidence supporting the belief that parenting has an important impact on mental health in adulthood is also strong. Whilst there are no intervention studies with very long-term follow-up, there are those which demonstrate a positive impact on the childhood antecedents of adult mental illness. The direct evidence that parenting has an impact on physical health in adulthood rests primarily on two studies. Both provide evidence which meets all the causality criteria apart from those requiring intervention studies with long-term follow-up. The research evidence that parenting has an impact on psychological health and emotional well-being in adolescence and adulthood, and that it also has an impact on unhealthy lifestyles, is the weakest of that presented in this chapter. It amounts to the demonstration of a statistical association in several studies, some of which adjust for confounding factors and some of which measure the putative cause before the putative effect.

The implications of this model for health and well-being are very great. The supporting research evidence is sufficiently strong to make the establishment of further studies something of a priority. Long-term follow-up studies are needed which are expensive and resource intensive. There are, however, intervention studies in progress at present which are funded to provide long-term follow-up and could be expanded to incorporate the essential range of outcome measures. Cohort studies are also being considered which could document parenting practices and parenting interventions in a way that is consistent with the evidence presented here about what is important in parent–child relationships. Future studies testing the importance of relationships at the centre of the model are likely to depend on the development of a range of widely accepted and validated measures of emotional well-being for children and adults. Other types of research design, for example qualitative and action research projects, will be needed to investigate the assertion that the development of social policy that supports the development of social well-being, depends on the emotional well-being of policy makers. An important factor determining whether any of these studies are set up will be the capacity of the research community and grant-giving bodies to entertain the possibility that children's emotional well-being could be this important for us all.

References

American Psychiatric Association (1987). *Diagnostic and statistical manual of mental disorders (DSM IV)*. Washington, DC, American Psychiatric Association.
Andrews, F. M. and Robinson, J. P. (1991). Measures of subjective well-being. In J. P. Robinson, P. R. Shaver and L. S. Wrightsman (eds.), *Measures of personality and social psychological attitudes*. San Diego, Academic, pp. 64–114.
Bardone, A. M., Moffitt, T. E., Caspi, A., *et al.* (1996). Adult mental health and social outcomes of adolescent girls with depression and conduct disorder. *Development and Psychopathology*, **8**, 811–29.
Barlow, J. and Stewart-Brown, S. (2000). Behaviour problems and parent education programmes. *Journal of Developmental and Behavioural Pediatrics*, 21(5).
Barnes, G. M. (1984). Adolescent alcohol abuse and other problem behaviour: their relationship and common parental influences. *Journal of Youth and Adolescence*, **13**, 329–84.

Baumrind, D. (1966). Effects of authoritative parental control on child behaviour. *Child Development*, **37**, 887–907.

Baumrind, D. (1971). Current patterns of parental authority. *Developmental Psychology Monograph*, **4**, 1–103.

Baumrind, D. (1978). Parental disciplinary patterns and social competence in children. *Youth and Society*, **9**, 239–75.

Baumrind, D. (1991). The influence of parenting style on adolescent competence and substance use. *Journal of Early Adolescence*, **11**, 56–9.

Becker, W. C. (1964). Consequences of different types of parental discipline. In M. L. Hoffman and L. Hoffman (eds.), *Review of child development research*, pp. 169–208. Vol. 1. New York, Sage.

Berkman, L. F. (1995). The role of social relations in health promotion. *Psychosomatic Research*, **57**, 245–54.

Berkman, L. F. and Syme, S. L. (1979). Social networks, host resistance and mortality: a nine year follow up of Alameda county residents. *American Journal of Epidemiology*, **109**, 186–204.

Blaxter, M. (1990). *Health and lifestyles*. London, Tavistock/Routledge.

Bruhn, J. G. and Wolf, S. (1979). *The Roseto story*. Norman, University of Oklahoma Press.

Brunner, E. (1997). Stress, biology and inequalities. *British Medical Journal*, **314**, 1472–6.

Capaldi, D. M., and Clark, S. (1998). Prospective family predictors of aggression toward female partners for young at-risk males. *Developmental Psychology*, **34**(6) 1175–88.

Capaldi, D. and Stoolmiller, M. (1999). Co-occurrence of conduct problems and depressive symptoms in early adolescent boys: III Prediction to young-adult adjustment. *Development and Psychopathology*, **11**(1), 59–84.

Caspi, A. and Silva, P. A. (1995). Temperamental qualities at age three predict personality traits in young adulthood: Longitudinal evidence from a birth cohort. *Child Development*, **66**, 486–98.

Caspi, A., Moffitt, T. E., Newman, D. L. and Silva, P. A. (1996). Behavioural observations at age 3 years predict adult psychiatric disorder. Longitudinal evidence from a birth cohort. *Archives of General Psychiatry*, **53**, 1033–9.

Caspi, A., Begg, D., Dickson, N., Langley. L., Moffit, T. E. and Silva, P. A. (1995). Identification of personality types at risk for poor health and injury in late adolescence. *Criminal Behaviour and Mental Health*, **5**, 330–50.

Ciliska, D., Hayward, J., Thomas, H., *et al.* (1994). *The effectiveness of home visiting as a delivery strategy for public health nursing interventions: a systematic review*. Working Paper Series 94–7. Hamilton, Ontario. McMaster University; Toronto University.

Cohen, D., Richardson, J. and Labree, L. (1994). Parenting behaviours and the onset of smoking and alcohol use: a longitudinal study. *Pediatrics*, **94**: 368–75.

Cohen, S. (1988). Psycho-social models of the role of social support in the aetiology of physical disease. *Health Psychology*, **7**, 269–97.

Davis, H. (1993). *Counselling parents of children with chronic illness or disability*. Leicester, BPS.

Dornbusch, S. Ritter, P. L., Leiberman, P. H. and Roberts, D. F. (1987). The relation of parenting style to adolescent school performance. *Child Development*, **58**, 1244–57.

Egan, G. (1982). *The skilled helper*. Monterey, CA, Brooks/Cole.

Farrington, D. P. (1994). Early developmental progression of juvenile delinquency. *Criminal Behaviour Mental Health*, **4**, 209–27.

Goleman, D. (1996). *Emotional intelligence*. London, Bloomsbury.

Goleman, D. (1998). *Working with emotional intelligence*. London, Bloomsbury.

Gordon, T. (1975). *Parent effectiveness training*. New York, Peter Wyden.

Gottman, J. and Declaire, J. (1997). *The heart of parenting: how to raise an emotionally intelligent child*. London, Bloomsbury.

Graves, P. L. (1991). Familial and psychological predictors of cancer. *Cancer Detection Preview*, **15**, 59–65.

Hoghughi, M. (1998). The importance of parenting in child health. *British Medical Journal*, **316**, 154.

Kelly, C. G. G. (1983). Adolescents' perception of three styles of parental control. *Adolescence*, **18**, 567–71.

LeShan, L. (1966). An emotional life-story pattern associated with neoplastic disease. *Annual New York Academic Science*, **125**, 780–93.

Loeber, R. (1983). Early predictors of male delinquency: a review. *Psychological Bulletin*, **94**, 68–99.

Loeber, R. and Dishion, T. (1997). Key issues in the development of aggression and violence from childhood to early adulthood. *Annual Review of Psychology*, **48**, 371–410.

Lundberg, O. (1993). The impact of childhood living conditions on illness and mortality in adulthood. *Social Sciences and Medicine*, **36**, 1047–52.

McClun, L. A. (1998). Relationship of perceived parenting styles, locus of control orientation and self-concept among junior high age students. *Psychology in the Schools*, **35**(4), 381–9.

McCord, W. (1963). Familial correlates of aggression in non delinquent male children. *Journal of Abnormal Social Psychology*, **62**, 72–93.

Moffit, T. E., Caspi, A., Dickson, N., *et al.* (1996). Childhood-onset versus adolescent-onset antisocial conduct problems in males. Natural history from ages 3–18 years. *Developmental Psychology*, **8**, 399–424.

Offord, D. R. and Bennett, K. J. (1994). Conduct disorder: long term outcomes and intervention effectiveness. *Journal of American Academy of Child Adolescent Psychiatry*, **33**, 1069–78.

Ornish, D. (1998). *Love and survival*. London, Vermilion.

Patterson, G. R. (1989). A developmental perspective on antisocial behaviour. *American Journal of Psychiatry*, **44**, 329–35.

Patterson, G. R., Dishion, T. J. and Chamberlain, P. (1993). Outcomes and methodological issues relating to the treatment of antisocial children. In T. R. Giles (ed.), *Handbook of effective psychotherapy*, pp. 43–89. New York, Plenum.

Pavis, S., Masters, H. and Cunningham Burley, S. (1996). *Lay concepts of positive mental health and how it can be maintained.* Edinburgh, University of Edinburgh Press.

Putnam, R. D., Leonardi, R. and Nanetti, R. Y. (1993). *Making democracy work: civic traditions in modern Italy.* Princetown, Princetown University Press.

Roberts, I., Kramer, M. S. and Suissa, S. (1996). Does home visiting prevent childhood injury. A systematic review of randomised controlled trials. *British Medical Journal*, **312**, 29–33.

Robins, L. N. (1981). Epidemiological approaches to natural history research: antisocial disorders in children. *Journal of American Academy of Child Psychiatry*, **20**, 566–680.

Rogers, C. (1959). A theory of therapy, personality and interpersonal relationships as developed in the client centred framework. In S. Koch (ed.), *Psychology: a study of science: formulations of the personal and social context*, pp. 184–256. Vol. 3. New York, McGraw-Hill.

Russek, L. G. and Schwartz, G. E. (1997a). Perceptions of parental caring predict health status in mid-life. *Psychosomatic Medicine*, **59**, 144–9.

Russek, L. G. and Schwartz, G. E. (1997b). Feelings of parental caring predict health status in midlife: a 35 year follow-up of the Harvard Mastery of Stress Study. *Journal of Behavioural Medicine*, **20**(1), 1–13.

Seeman, T. E. and Syme, L. (1987). Social networks and coronary artery disease: a comparison of the structure and function of social relations as predictors of disease. *Psychosomatic Medicine*, **49**, 341–54.

Smith, C. (1996). *Developing parenting programmes.* London, National Children's Bureau.

Steinberg, L., Elmen, J. D. and Mounts, N. S. (1989). Authoritative parenting, psycho-social maturity, and academic success among adolescents. *Child Development*, **60**, 1424–36.

Steiner, C. (1997). *Achieving emotional literacy.* London, Bloomsbury.

Stewart, M. A. (1985). Aggressive conduct disorder: a brief review. Sixth Biennial Meeting of the International Society for Research on Aggression. *Aggressive Behaviour*, **11**, 323–31.

Stone, D., Patton, B. and Heen, S. (1999). *Difficult conversations.* London, Michael Joseph.

Tudor, K. (1996). *Mental health promotion: paradigms and practice.* London, Routledge.

Utting, D., Bright, J. and Henricson, C. (1993). Crime and the family:

improving child rearing and preventing delinquency. *Occasional Paper 16*. London, Family Policy Studies Centre.
Weare, K. (2000). *Promoting mental emotional and social health: a whole school approach*. London, Routledge.
Webster-Stratton, C. (1999). Researching the impact of parent training programmes on child conduct disorder. In E. Loyd (ed.), *What works in parenting education*, pp. 85–114. Barkingside: Barnado's.
Wilkinson, R. G. (1996). *Unhealthy societies: the afflictions of inequality*. London and New York, Routledge.
World Health Organisation (1947). The Constitution of the World Health Organisation. *WHO Chronicle*. Vol. 1. Geneva, World Health Organisation.
World Health Organisation (1986). The Ottawa Charter for health promotion. *International Conference on Health Promotion*. Ottawa, World Health Organisation.

Notes

1. Strong and consistent relationship which persists after adjustment for confounding factors; evidence of a dose–response relationship; evidence that the putative cause precedes the putative effect; and evidence that interventions which impact on the putative cause have an impact on the putative effect.

3

In and out of emotional and behavioural problems

Eirini Flouri, Ann Buchanan, and Victoria Bream

'Many difficult children become less difficult with age, and a minority of very difficult children become apparently normal adults. The natural histories of children who turn out to be normal adults despite the serious behavioural problems that generally predict adult difficulty are of great interest because they reveal environmental interventions or concurrent personality traits and skills that seem to counterbalance the bad prognosis associated with this behaviour.' **Robins and Rutter 1990, p. xiv**

Since Rutter and his colleagues' study in the Isle of Wight (1970), further studies from around the world have tried to quantify the number of maladjusted children. These early studies give the numbers of children with significant problems *at one point of time*, be it in a community or in a wider population. They tell us little about what happens to the children *over* time.

With the development of the longitudinal studies, especially the large national birth cohort studies, it became possible to plot the natural histories of children. Initially, these longitudinal studies painted a rather depressing picture of 'continuity' of maladjustment problems from childhood to adult life. Less attention was paid to 'discontinuity', or those young people who 'recovered' and became apparently normal adults.

This chapter reports the findings of a recently completed study using data from the National Child Development Study (NCDS). This study shows that half of all children who had significant emotional and behavioural problems at one age, did not at another – that is, they 'came through' or 'recovered', and only 9% of the children who had problems in childhood went on to experience psychological problems in early adult life. To be 'effective', interventions must improve on the progress that most of these children will achieve in the natural course of events.

The prevalence of maladjustment

Depending on the age of the child, the area in which he or she lives, their sex, the time period, the specific type of disorder and the method of assessment, the prevalence of maladjustment ranges from 6% to 25%. Rutter *et al.* (1970) in the Isle of Wight found an overall prevalence of emotional and behavioural disorders of 7% at ages 10 and 11. When that study was repeated in inner London, the rates were more than doubled. The prevalence of a disorder was 25% for boys and 13% for girls (Rutter *et al.* 1975).

Gould *et al.* (1981), in a review of 25 American and British studies, gave an overall figure of 16% as a conservative estimate of prevalence of all disorders at ages 10 and 11. Anderson *et al.* (1987), in a study of 792 children aged 11 years from the general population in New Zealand, found an overall prevalence of disorder of 18% with a sex ratio (boys : girls) of 1.7 : 1. However, these authors suggest that if the term 'disorder' is limited to those children whose problems are pervasive, the prevalence drops to 7%.

As can be seen from Table 3.1, studies examining the prevalence of maladjustment have used a range of assessment tools. Most scales, including the Rutter scales, define their problem groups on the basis of a cut-off score on checklist measures. The prevalence varies depending on whether the informant is a parent, a teacher or the child him/herself. For example, in Rutter's checklists, Rutter 'A' is the parent report and Rutter 'B' the teacher report. There are no Rutter checklists for children, but more recently Goodman (1994) has developed from the original Rutter scales the Strengths and Difficulties Questionnaire which now includes a child report scale. Ideally, children's adjustment should be assessed from multi-sources.

Table 3.1 Some key prevalence studies

Study	Size	Age	Method	Definition	Assessment method	Prevalence
Davie et al. 1972, UK	15 039	7	Whole birth cohort	Arbitrary cut-off on teacher's scale; parents' scale individual problems	BSAG: parent questionnaire	14%
Fogelman 1976, UK	11 692	16	Whole birth cohort	Individual problems	Rutter A/B	N.A.
Fombonne 1994, Chartres, France	2441	6–11	2-stage; children from random schools; over-sampling special classes	Clinical/statistical	CBCL; Rutter B; Rutter and Graham parent interview; CGAS	12.4%
Glow 1978, Adelaide, Australia	2475	Grade k-6	Random urban schools	Statistical	Conners' Teacher Rating scale	29% significant 9.8% teacher-rated severe
Graham and Rutter 1973, Isle of Wight	2303	14–15	Total population; 2-stage	Clinical	Rutter A/B; Rutter parent/child/teacher interview	Boys 13.2%; girls 12.5%
Kellam et al. 1975, Chicago, USA	2010	Gr 1. F-Up Gr. 3	Population: 1-graders, poor, urban	Teachers' perception/ mother's ratings/ clinical judgement	Questionnaires for teachers, mothers, observers, child	19.4% moderately 13.6% severely maladapted
Koot and Verhulst 1991, The Netherlands	420	2–3	Random selection	Statistical/individual problems	CBCL	12.6%

Study	N	Age	Sample	Judgement	Assessment	Results
Langner et al. 1976, New York, USA	1034	6–18	Random sample households	Statistical and clinical judgement	Parent questionnaire/child interview	13% with disorder
Leslie 1974, UK	1198	13–14	Total population in secondary school. 2-stage	Clinical	Parent/teacher; Rutter parent/child interviews	17.2% Boys 21%, girls 14%
Matsuura et al. 1993, Japan	2638	6–12	Children in primary school	Statistical	Rutter A/B	Parents 12%; teachers 3.9%
Matsuura et al. 1993, China	2432	6–12	Children in primary school	Statistical	Rutter A/B	Parents 7%; teachers 8.3%
Matsuura et al. 1993, Korea	1975	6–12	Children in primary school	Statistical	Rutter A/B	Parents 19.1%; teachers 14.1%
McGee et al. 1984, Dunedin, NZ	951	7	Total sample born in one hospital	Statistical	Rutter A/B during psychometric assessment	30% high level of problem behaviours
Miller et al. 1974, Newcastle-upon-Tyne, UK	2615	10	Whole birth cohort using household census	Impairment; rating by parent and interviewer	Parent/school information	19.4% maladjusted
Morita et al. 1993, Japan	1992	12–15	Children in secondary schools; 2-stage	Statistical/clinical	Rutter A/B; Rutter child interview	16% 12–13 years 14% 14–15 years
Oliver 1974, USA	6768	12–17	Random sample of national population	Teachers' perception of emotional adjustment	Teacher questionnaire	Boys 18.7%; girls 12.3%; 75% well-adjusted
Rahim and Cederblad 1984, Sudan	8462	3–15	Whole population of 3 villages; 2-stage	Individual problems/ clinical judgement	Parent questionnaire/ parent interview	13% severe; 47% problem free

Table 3.1 – *continued*

Study	Size	Age	Method	Definition	Assessment method	Prevalence
Rutter *et al.* 1970, Isle of Wight, UK	3316	10–11	Total island public school population; 2- stage	Clinical	Rutter A/B; Rutter parent/child interview	6.8% excluding mental retardation
Rutter *et al.* 1975, Inner London	1689	10	Total population of children in LA schools; 2-stage	Clinical	Rutter B, Rutter parent interview	25.4%
Werner *et al.* 1971, Hawaii, USA	750	10	Household census pregnant women; child follow-up	Interference with school achievement and individual items	Home interview/ teacher questionnaire	26%: 1+ problems; 1 in 6 had problems affecting school

Source: based on Verhulst and Koot 1975.

Internalising versus externalising disorders

Types of maladjustment in children are often broadly categorised as 'internalising' and 'externalising' disorders. 'Internalising' refers to conditions whose central feature is disordered emotion. In contrast, 'externalising disorders' are those whose central feature is dysregulated behaviour. The terms 'emotional' versus 'behavioural' disorders are broadly synonymous with 'internalising' versus 'externalising' conditions (Kovacs and Devlin 1998). Within these two broad groups, there are a number of sub-groups. Internalising disorders comprise both depressive and anxiety disorders. Similarly, 'externalising' disorders also have a number of sub-categories, for example, Attention Deficit Hyperactive Disorder, Oppositional Defiant Disorder, and Conduct Disorder (American Psychiatric Association 1987).

There is a continuing debate about co-morbidity. Throughout childhood and adolescence internalising disorders are more likely to be co-morbid with one another (for example anxiety and depression) than with externalising disorders (Cohen *et al.* 1993; Hewitt *et al.* 1997). Internalising disorders, however, co-occur with externalising disorders at rates typically higher than by chance (Caron and Rutter 1991). Children with externalising disorders may develop depression in adult life (Eaves *et al.* 1997). Those with internalising disorders may progress from anxiety to early childhood behaviour problems and then to depression (Kovacs and Devlin 1998).

Evaluations from longitudinal data in New Zealand at ages 15, 18, and 21 demonstrate that all internalising disorders occur at a lower rate in childhood than in adolescence or adulthood. For example, the prevalence of anxiety disorder rises from 8% at 11 to 19% at 21, and of depressive disorder from 1.8% at 11 to 19% at 21. Externalising disorders presented a rather different picture; they rise from 9% at 11 to 12% at age 15 and they drop to 6% at age 18 (McGee *et al.* 1990; Feehan *et al.* 1994; Newman *et al.* 1996). There is considerable agreement that while externalising disorders are more usual amongst boys, internalising disorders are more common amongst girls although there are disorder-specific age trends (Hewitt *et al.* 1997).

Stability of childhood problems

Kovacs and Devlin (1998) note that findings from epidemiological, community-based, clinically referred and special samples
converge in supporting the predictive validity of internalising
disorders in the younger years from childhood to adolescence to
adulthood. Similarly, findings from children with externalising
disorders paint a rather depressing picture of continuity from
childhood into adult life (Robins 1991; Campbell 1995). Robins
notes that most children with pervasive disorders at 13 could
have been identified as demonstrating 'externalising' behaviours
as early as at 3 years old:

Eighty-four per cent of children found to be 'uncontrolled' at age 11
met criteria for stable and pervasive antisocial disorder when reassessed
at 13. Antisocial behaviour at 13 was predicted by 'externalising'
behaviour at 3 and behaviour problems at 5, long before a diagnosis of
conduct disorder could be made. Further, these early behaviours were
stronger predictors than high non-verbal skills, mothers' attitudes,
language level or any other variable tested. (Robins 1991, p. 202.)

Similarly, most children with later depression have exhibited
an anxiety-type disorder earlier in childhood:

The weight of evidence that youngsters with emotional disorders are
likely to have similar difficulties in young adulthood will presumably
put to rest any lingering notions that depressive or anxiety disorders in
young people are a temporary phase. (Kovacs and Devlin 1998, p. 51.)

Despite this evidence of 'stability' in disorders throughout
childhood, the same results can often show 'recovery' (Campbell
1995; Kovacs and Devlin 1998). Campbell's conclusion that half
of 3-year-olds with hard-to-manage behaviour go on to have
later difficulties also means that half do not. Although there is an
impressive body of evidence from longitudinal studies of continuity of antisocial behaviour throughout childhood, results also
show a substantial element of discontinuity.

Similarly, Kovacs and Devlin's (1998) conclusion that environmental factors, perhaps in combination with 'within-person'
factors, account for the heterogeneity of outcomes for children
with internalising disorders gives the hope that within the
broader 'ecology' (family, school, neighbourhood) of the envi-

ronment in which children are brought up (Bronfenbrenner 1979), it may be possible to identify protective factors or compensatory experiences for children who not have them naturally (Rutter 1995).

Kazdin (1995), in a major review of studies on conduct disorder, notes that much less is known about protective factors than about risk factors. He suggests that evaluation of protective factors warrants much further work because fostering these factors represents a viable approach to the prevention of conduct disorder.

Similarly, when considering internalising disorders, Fombonne (1995) suggests that one of the most important issues on the research agenda is the identification of protective mechanisms for those at risk that help build healthy developmental pathways into adult life.

Koot (1995), in an overview of longitudinal studies of the general population and community samples, reports on a number of studies that consider stability and change in children with emotional and behavioural disorders over time. Across the studies, one third to one half of children having initial deviant scores maintain scores across the 2- to 6-year intervals.

- In the Zuid-Holland study the 2-, 4-, and 6-year stability of parent-report problem behaviours, as well as teacher- and adolescent-report, was noted in a sample of 2076 children aged between 4 and 16 years. Using standardised measurements (Achenbach and Edelbrock 1983), Pearson correlations for the stability of parent-rated problems scores were 0.67, 0.63, and 0.56 across the 2-, 4-, and 6-year intervals, respectively.
- Ghodsian *et al.* (1980), using data from the 17 000 children involved in the NCDS and different instruments at different ages, found correlations for parent ratings of 0.48 between 7 and 11 years, 0.38 between 7 and 16 years, and 0.46 between 11 and 16 years.
- The Berkeley Growth Study (MacFarlane *et al.* 1962), involving a much smaller group of children (*n* = 116) followed children over 14 years with follow-up sweeps every 18 months. Correlations for total problem scores averaged around 0.52 for boys and 0.45 for girls.

- Koot (1995) noted that in the Zuid-Holland study, of the children who were in the deviant range of the total problem score at time 1, 54%, 44%, and 33% were scored deviant after 2, 4, and 6 years, respectively.

The current study – 'recovery' from emotional and behavioural problems.

The aim of the study was, using longitudinal data from the NCDS, to track children who had moderate or severe emotional and behavioural problems (EBPs) at age 7, and/or 11, and/or 16 into adulthood age 33. The purpose was to assess the numbers who 'recovered', that is, did not fall into the top 20% band of children with problems at the next measurement point and who did not have psychological problems at age 33.

The data was derived from sweeps of the NCDS. The NCDS has tracked 17 000 children born between 3 and 9 March 1958 in England, Scotland, and Wales. Five follow-ups were carried out: in 1965 (age 7); in 1969 (age 11); in 1974 (age 16); in 1981 (age 23) and in 1991 (age 33).

The psychological measures used in this study

All the childhood emotional and behavioural measures in this study were based on the Rutter A Health and Behaviour Checklist. Since its development in the Isle of Wight study (Rutter *et al.* 1970) as discussed earlier, the Rutter A has been widely used for research and translated for many studies around the world. Generally, a cut-off score of 13+ is used to identify a significant level of maladjustment, but, as we have seen, the number of children who fall into this category differs by age, gender, and area.

Goodman (1994), in developing the Strengths and Difficulties Questionnaire, argues that a better strategy for researchers is a percentage cut-off. For his questionnaire, bands are chosen so that, roughly, 80% of children are normal, 10% are borderline, and 10% are abnormal.

In this study, a similar strategy has been used. It was felt that a 20% cut-off of the highest scores best identified the top range of children with the more difficult behaviour at each age.

The adult psychological measures are based on the Malaise Inventory. At age 33 cohort members in the study were asked to complete this checklist. This inventory is a 24-item list of symptoms from the Cornell Medical Index, developed by the Institute of Psychiatry. A score of 8+ on the inventory has been widely used to identify those at risk of depression (Richman 1978; Pound *et al.* 1988; Thorpe *et al.* 1991). Of the 6441 people about whom there were complete psychological measures at all ages, 414 (6%) had a Malaise score of 8 or greater at age 33. This percentage compares well with that from an earlier study using the NCDS (Buchanan and Ten Brinke 1997), in which 7.6% of the much larger sample involved had high Malaise scores at age 33.

Development of the emotional and behavioural scores

In the NCDS, emotional and behavioural measures were taken at age 7, 11, and 16 years. In 1974 at age 16 the full Rutter A (31 questions) Health and Behaviour Checklist was completed by the parent or primary care giver. At both age 7 (1965) and 11 (1969) a shortened parental version was used. Researchers have used variants of this shorter Rutter A (e.g. Elliott and Richards 1991; Chase-Lansdale *et al.* 1995).

Twenty-three items from the Rutter A Health and Behaviour Checklist were available at all three ages, 7, 11, and 16. As in Silberg *et al.*'s (1996) study, which used the full Rutter A, factor analysis on these 23 items at age 16 showed that two sets of behaviours grouped together, forming an 'internalising' group and an 'externalising' group (a third group related to health problems). This shortened Rutter A was subsequently compared with the full Rutter A at age 16 and it was found that the two were highly correlated ($r = 0.95$, $p < 0.001$). Similarly, a 20% cut-off applied to both the shortened and the full Rutter A largely identified the same individuals (chi-square = 2841.45, df:1, $p = 0.001$).

The 20% cut-off for each age (7, 11, and 16) shifted marginally depending on how the numbers fell into each score.

Development of the 'internalising' and the 'externalising' subgroups

The 'internalising' and 'externalising' scores were calculated from the total score for each response. Scoring procedures for assessing the internalising and externalising groups replicated those used for the full Rutter A. The factor analysis carried out to explore the dimensionality of the Rutter A in this sample showed that the 'internalising' subgroup was based on the total score for positive responses to having headaches, stomach-aches, sleep problems, worries, and being solitary, miserable, and fearful. The 'externalising' subgroup was based on the total score for positive responses to being fidgety, destroying things, fighting, not being liked and being irritable, disobedient, and unsettled.

To check the validity of these subgroups, the 'externalising' and 'internalising' subgroups were compared to the subgroups of the full Rutter A at 16. As mentioned above, the short and long versions of the Rutter A at age 16 showed a good correlation. The continuous measure for the subgroup 'internalising' from the short Rutter A was compared to the continuous measure for the subgroup 'neurotic' on the full Rutter A ($r = 0.80$, $p < 0.001$). Similarly, the continuous measure for the subgroup 'externalising' from the short Rutter A was compared to 'conduct disorder' on the full Rutter A ($r = 0.61$, $p < 0.001$).

Children with an 'internalising' score exceeding their 'externalising' score were designated as having an 'internalising' problem, while those with an 'externalising' score exceeding their 'internalising' score were designated as having an 'externalising' problem. Children who had equal internalising and externalising scores (the co-morbid group) were omitted from the subgroup analyses but not from the group analyses. A total of 293 children (5%) of the sample fell into the co-morbid group at one or more of the time periods (7, 11, 16).

The findings

Table 3.2 shows the numbers and percentages of children who had EBPs at one age (7, 11, 16) and a high Malaise score at age 33, and those who had EBPs and a high Malaise score at multiple ages.

The first striking impression is that just under half of the sample had EBPs or a high Malaise score at some age between 7 and 33. This finding suggests that psychological problems, in childhood and adult life, as defined here, involve substantial numbers of children and young people. In this study we were looking at children with both borderline and severe EBPs. It is likely that had we just considered significant EBPs (or the top 10%), our figures would have been nearer to those of McGee *et al.* (1995) who found that over the period from pre-school to pre-adolescent years around 25% of children had a significant mental health problem.

The positive finding from our study was that of the 6641 children in the sample, 56% did not have EBPs (as defined) in childhood nor mental health problems in adulthood, and only 51 people (1%) had EBPs at all three ages in childhood and psychological problems in adulthood. A quarter of the sample (25%) had a mental health problem at one age only, 12% had a problem at two age points, and only 6% had a problem at three age points. These initial findings seem to suggest that there is considerable entry into and exit out of EBPs.

Internalising and externalising problems

As might be expected, there appeared to be an excess of boys over girls with externalising problems at 7 and 11. By the same token, there appeared to be an excess of girls over boys with internalising problems at 11. By the age of 16 this gap widened, with around 16% of girls falling into the top band of internalising scores compared to 11% of boys. These figures, however, were a little confounded because around 2% at each age fell into a co-morbid group; that is their internalising and externalising scores were equal.

Table 3.2 People with psychological problems at single or multiple time points by gender

	All	Percentage	Female	Percentage	Male	Percentage
	6441	100	3326	100	3115	100
No problems (Neither EBPs at 7, 11, or 16, nor Malaise at 33)	3577	56	1812	55	1765	57
Problems at one age only						
7	545	8	249	7	296	9
11	381	6	177	5	204	7
16	552	8	322	10	230	7
33	171	3	116	4	55	2
Total	1649	25	864	26	785	25
Problems at two ages						
7, 11	210	3	85	3	125	4
7, 16	210	3	117	3	93	3
7, 33	36	1	25	1	11	1
11, 16	228	4	124	4	104	3
11, 33	25	0	15	0	10	0
16, 33	53	1	44	1	9	0
Total	762	12	410	12	352	11
Problems at three ages						
7, 11, 16	324	5	156	5	168	5
7, 11, 33	18	0	11	0	7	0
7, 16, 33	22	0	19	0	3	0
11, 16, 33	38	1	27	1	11	1
Total	402	6	213	6	189	6
Problems at all ages						
7, 11, 16, 33	51	1	27	1	24	1

Recovery and stability

Looking at Table 3.3, one can see that of the 7-year-olds with EBPs 43% went on to have problems when they were aged 11, and 43% of those who had problems at 11 had difficulties when they were 16 years old. Similarly, of the 11-year-olds with EBPs 50% went on to have problems at age 16. These findings loosely approximate those reported in McGee *et al.* (1992), who found that 40% of those children with a disorder at age 11 were also identified as having that disorder at 15. These findings suggest that at least half of children with mental health problems at each age 'recover'.

Looking at the other side of the coin, one can also argue that there seems to be overall psychological stability across ages. For example, externalising scores at age 7 were significantly correlated with externalising scores at 11 ($r = 0.43$, $p < 0.001$), and 16 ($r = 0.33$, $p < 0.001$), and externalising scores at 11 were positively correlated with externalising scores at 16 ($r = 0.42$, $p < 0.001$). By the same token, internalising scores at age 7 were positively related to internalising scores at ages 11 ($r = 0.31$, $p < 0.001$) and 16 ($r = 0.15$, $p < 0.001$), and internalising scores at age 11 correlated positively with internalising scores at age 16 ($r = 0.37$, $p < 0.001$).

These findings compare well with the correlations reported in other studies. For example, Ghodsian *et al.* (1980), also using NCDS data but different instruments at different ages and focussing on the top 13% 'deviant' group at each age, found overall stability for parent ratings of 0.48 between the ages of 7 and 11, 0.46 between 11 and 16, and 0.38 between 7 and 16.

Table 3.3 Occurrence of EBPs across ages

	EBPs at 7	EBPs at 11	EBPs at 16
EBPs at 7 ($n = 1416$)	–	603 (43%)*	607 (43%)*
EBPs at 11 ($n = 1275$)	603 (43%)*	–	641** (50%)
EBPs at 16 ($n = 1478$)	607 (43%)*	641** (50%)	–

* Percentage based on those with EBPs at 7.
** Percentage based on those with EBPs at 11.

Similar findings are reported in MacFarlane *et al.* (1962) who took yearly measurements. From birth to 14 years, the correlations between total problem scores averaged 0.52 for boys and 0.45 for girls. As in this study, correlations decreased with increasing time intervals between measurements.

Continuity and discontinuity

Striking differences are seen depending upon whether the data is viewed retrospectively or prospectively (see Tables 3.4 and 3.5). Looking *back* in time from when the cohort members were 33 years old, one can see that 31% of all individuals with a high Malaise score at 33 also had EBPs, as defined, at age 7, which indicates a considerable *continuity* of psychological problems between childhood and adulthood (see Table 3.4). On the other hand, looking *forward* from when the cohort members were 7 years old, one can see that only 9% of all those individuals who had EBPs at age 7 went on to have a high Malaise score at age 33, which indicates considerable *discontinuity* of mental health problems between childhood and adulthood (see Table 3.5).

In part, these figures reflect how the psychological problems in childhood were defined in this study and the numbers involved. The point needs to be made, however, lest we forget when we see that nearly a third of those with a high Malaise score in adult life had emotional and behavioural problems in childhood, that 91% of children who had EBPs in childhood did *not* go on to have psychological difficulties in adult life.

Table 3.4 Looking back from age 33

	EBPs at 7 (n = 1416)	No EBPs at 7 (n = 5025)	Total
High Malaise at 33 (n = 414)	127 (31% of high Malaise group)	287 (69% of high Malaise group)	414
Low Malaise at 33 (n = 6027)	1289	4738	6027
Total	1416	5025	6441

Table 3.5 Looking forward from age 7

	High Malaise at 33 (*n* = 414)	Low Malaise at 33 (*n* = 6027)	Total
EBPs at 7 (*n* = 1416)	127 (9% of those with EBPs at 7)	1289 (91% of those with EBPs at 7)	1416
No EBPs at 7 (*n* = 5025)	287	4738	5025
Total	414	6027	6441

Discussion

This study was carried out to explore stability and change in children with emotional and behavioural disorders over time. The findings described above suggest that a large number of children have borderline or significant EBPs in childhood, and that these problems link with adult mental health. Forty-five per cent of the sample had mental health problems at some stage between ages 7 and 33. Such problems are likely to impinge on educational and career opportunities, affect health, and probably affect relationships. If such problems can be prevented, it is likely to be of benefit not only to the individual and society, but may also ease the pressures on the NHS budget.

The encouraging finding is that large numbers of children 'recover'. At each age, the recovery rate is around 50% and more than a quarter of the cohort members (26%) with mental health problems had these at one age only.

We need to bear in mind, however, that this 'recovery' rate may be overestimated in this study. These findings are likely to be affected by bias due to attrition and/or missing data. Analyses of missing data from the NCDS and other mental health studies (Cox *et al.* 1977; Buchanan and Ten Brinke 1997) suggest that precisely those individuals about whom we have incomplete information are more likely to experience poorer outcomes. Our findings, therefore, are likely to underestimate the occurrence of psychological problems particularly at age 16 and in adult life when the attrition rates were highest.

Nevertheless, these findings give hope for clinicians and others who seek to help children with emotional and behavioural problems that 'recovery' is possible. The challenge is to elicit the mechanisms associated with this recovery, and to develop effective programmes, so that affected children can be helped to overcome their difficulties.

Acknowledgements

This study was undertaken by Ann Buchanan, JoAnn Ten Brinke, and Eirini Flouri, who received funding from the NHS Executive Anglia and Oxford; the views expressed in this chapter are those of the authors and not necessarily those of the NHS Executive Anglia and Oxford.

References

Achenbach, T. M. and Edelbrock, C. (1983). *Manual for the child behavior checklist and revised child behavior profile*. Burlington, VT, Department of Psychiatry, University of Vermont,..

American Psychiatric Association (1987). *Diagnostic and statistical manual of mental disorders*, 3rd edn – revised (DSM III-R). Washington, DC, American Psychiatric Association.

Anderson, J. C., Williams, S., McGee, R., and Silva, P. A. (1987). DSM-III disorders in preadolescent children: prevalence in a large sample from the general population. *Archives of General Psychiatry*, **44**, 69–76.

Bronfenbrenner, U. (1979). *The ecology of human development: experiments by nature and design*. Cambridge, MA, Harvard University Press.

Buchanan, A. and Ten Brinke, J. (1997). *What happened when they were grown up: Outcomes from parenting experiences*. York, Joseph Rowntree Foundation

Campbell, S. B. (1995). Behavior problems in preschool children: a review of recent research. *Journal of Child Psychology and Psychiatry*, **36**, 115–49.

Caron, C. and Rutter, M. (1991). Co-morbidity in child psychopathology: concepts, issues, and research strategies. *Journal of Child Psychology and Psychiatry*, **32**, 1063–80.

Chase-Lansdale, P. L., Cherlin, A. J., and Kiernan, K. E. (1995). The long-term effects of parental divorce on the mental health of young adults: a developmental perspective. *Child Development*, **66**, 1614–34.

Cohen, P., Cohen, J., Kasen, S., *et al.* (1993). An epidemiological study of disorders in late childhood and adolescence: I. Age- and gender-specific prevalence. *Journal of Child Psychology and Psychiatry*, **34**(6), 851–8.

Cox, A., Rutter, M., Yule, B., and Quinton, D. (1977). Bias resulting from missing information: some epidemiological findings. *Journal of Epidemiology and Community Health*. **31**, 131–6.

Davie, R., Butler, H., and Goldstein, H. (1972) *From birth to seven: the second report of the National Child Development Study (1958 cohort)*. Longman, London.

Eaves, L. J., Silberg, J. L., Simonoff, E., *et al.* (1997). Genetics and developmental psychopathology: 1. Phenotypic assessment in the Virginia twin study of adolescent behavioural assessment. *Journal of Child Psychology and Psychiatry*, **38**, 965–80.

Elliott, B. J. and Richards, M. (1991). Children and divorce: educational performance and behaviour before and after parental separation. *International Journal of Law and the Family*, **5**, 258–76.

Feehan, M., McGee, R., Raja, S. N., and Williams, S. M. (1994). DSM III-R disorders in New Zealand 18 year olds. *Australian and New Zealand Journal of Psychiatry*, **28**, 87–99.

Ferri, E. (1993). *Life at 33: the fifth follow-up of the National Child Development Study.* London, National Children's Bureau, City University, Economic and Social Research Council.

Fogelman, K. (1976). *Britain's sixteen-year-olds: Preliminary findings from the third follow-up of the National Child Development Study (1958 cohort)*. London, National Children's Bureau.

Fombonne, E. (1994). The Chartres study: prevalence of psychiatric disorders among French school-aged children. *British Journal of Psychiatry*, **164**, 69–79.

Fombonne, E. (1995). Depressive disorders: time trends and possible explanatory mechanisms. In M. Rutter and D. Smith (eds.), *Psychosocial disorders in young people*. Chichester, Wiley, pp. 544–615.

Ghodsian, M., Fogelman, K., Lambert, L., and Tibbenham, A. (1980). Changes in behaviour of a national sample of children. *British Journal of Social and Clinical Psychology*, **19**, 247–56.

Glow, R. A. (1978). *Classroom behaviour problems: an Australian normative study of Conners' Teacher Rating Scale*. University of Adelaide, Department of Psychology, Adelaide, Australia.

Goodman, R. (1994). A modified version of the Rutter parent questionnaire including extra items on children's strengths: a research note. *Journal of Child Psychology and Psychiatry*, **35**, 1483–94.

Gould, M. S., Wuch-Hitzig, R., and Dohrenwend, B. (1981). Estimating the prevalence of childhood psychopathology: a critical review. *Journal of the American Academy of Child and Adolescent Psychiatry*, **20**, 462–76.

Graham, P. and Rutter, M. (1973). Psychiatric disorder in the young adolescent: a follow-up study. *Proceedings of the Royal Society of Medicine*, **66**, 1226–8.

Hewitt, J. K., Eaves, L. J., Silberg, J. L., *et al.* (1997). Genetics and developmental psychopathology: 1. Phenotypic assessment in the Virginia twin study of adolescent behavioural assessment. *Journal of Child Psychology and Psychiatry*, **38**, 943–63.

Kazdin, A. E. (1995). Conduct disorder. In F. C. Verhulst and H. M. Koot (eds.), *The epidemiology of child and adolescent psychopathology*. Oxford, Oxford University Press, pp. 258–290.

Kellam, G. S., Branch, J. D., Agrawal, K. C., and Ensminger, M. E. (1975). *Mental health and going to school: the Woodlawn program of assessment, early intervention, and evaluation*. Chicago, IL, University of Chicago Press.

Koot, H. M. (1995). Longitudinal studies of general population and community samples. In F. C. Verhulst and H. M. Koot (eds.), *The epidemiology of child and adolescent psychopathology*. Oxford, Oxford University Press, pp. 337–365.

Koot, H. M. and Verhulst, F. C. (1991). Prevalence of problem behaviour in Dutch children age 2–3. *Acta Psychiatrica Scandinavica*, 83 (Suppl. 367).

Kovacs, M. and Devlin, B. (1998). Internalizing disorders in childhood. *Journal of Child Psychology and Psychiatry*, **39**, 47–63.

Langner, T. S., Gersten, J. C., McCarty, E. D., *et al.* (1976). A screening inventory for assessing psychiatric impairment in children 6 to 18. *Journal of Consulting and Clinical Psychology*, **44**, 286–96.

Leslie, S. A. (1974). Psychiatric disorder in the young adolescents of an industrial town. *British Journal of Psychiatry*, **125**, 113–24.

MacFarlane, J. W., Allen, L., and Honzik, M. P. (1962). *A developmental study of behaviour problems of normal children between twenty-one months and fourteen years*. Berkeley, CA, University of California Press.

Matsuura, M., Okubo, Y., Kato, M., Kojima, T. *et al.* (1993). A cross-national prevalence study of children with emotional and behavioural problems: a WHO collaborative study in the Western Pacific Region. *Journal of Child Psychology and Psychiatry*, **34**, 307–15.

McGee, R., Williams, S., and Silva, P. A. (1984). Behavioral and developmental characteristics of aggressive, hyperactive and aggressive-hyperactive boys. *Journal of the American Academy of Child and Adolescent Psychiatry*, **23**, 270–9.

McGee, R., Feehan, M., Williams, S., *et al.* (1990). DSM III disorders in a large sample of adolescents. *Journal of the American Academy of Child and Adolescent Psychiatry*, **29**, 611–19.

McGee, R., Feehan, M., Williams, S., and Anderson, J. (1992). DSM-III disorders from age 11 to age 15 years. *Journal of the American Academy of Child and Adolescent Psychiatry*, **31**, 50–9.

McGee, R., Feehan, M., and Williams, S. (1995). Long-term follow-up of a birth cohort. In F. C. Verhulst and H. M. Koot (eds.), *The epidemiology of child and adolescent psychopathology.* Oxford, Oxford University Press, pp. 366–84.

Miller, F. J. W., Court, S. D. M., Knox, E. G., and Brandon, S. (1974). *The school years in Newcastle upon Tyne 1952–62: being a further contribution to the study of a thousand families.* Oxford, Oxford University Press.

Morita, H., Suzuki, M., Suzuki, S., and Kamoshita, S. (1993). Psychiatric disorders in Japanese secondary school children. *Journal of Child Psychology and Psychiatry,* **34**, 317–32.

Newman, D. L., Moffitt, T. E., Caspi, A., *et al.* (1996). Psychiatric disorder in a birth cohort of young adults: prevalence, comorbidity, clinical significance and new case incidence from age 11 to 21. *Journal of Consulting and Clinical Psychology,* **64**, 552–62.

Offord, D. R., Boyle, M. H., Szatmari, P., *et al.* (1987). Ontario Child Health Study II: six-month prevalence of disorder and rates of service utilization. *Archives of General Psychiatry,* **44**, 832–6.

Oliver, L. I. (1974). *Behavior patterns in school of youths 12–17.* Washington, DC, Government Printing Office, DHEW Publication No. HRA 74–1621.

Pound, A., Puckering, C., Cox, T., and Mills, M. (1988). The impact of maternal depression on young children. *British Journal of Psychotherapy,* **4**, 240–52.

Rahim, S. I. and Cederblad, M. (1984). Effects of rapid urbanization on child behaviour and health in a part of Khartoum, Sudan. *Journal of Child Psychology and Psychiatry,* **25**, 629–41.

Richman, N. (1978). Depression in mothers of young children. *Journal of the Royal Society of Medicine,* **71**, 489–93.

Robins, L. N. (1991). Conduct disorder. *Journal of Child Psychology and Psychiatry,* **32**, 193–212.

Robins, L. N. and Rutter, M. (1990). Introduction. In L. Robins and M. Rutter (eds.), *Straight and devious pathways from childhood to adulthood.* Cambridge, Cambridge University Press, pp. xiii–xix.

Rutter, M. (1995). Causal concepts and their testing. In M. Rutter and D. Smith (eds.), *Psychosocial disorders in young people.* Chichester, Wiley, pp. 7–34.

Rutter, M., Tizard, J., and Whitmore, K. (1970). *Education, health and behaviour.* London, Longman.

Rutter, M., Cox, A., Tupling, C., Burger, M. and Yule, W. (1975). Attainment and adjustment in two geographical areas: I The prevalence of psychiatric disorder. *British Journal of Psychiatry,* **126**, 493–509.

Shepherd, P. (1993). Appendix I: Analysis of response bias. In E. Ferri (ed.), *Life at 33.* London, National Children's Bureau, pp. 184–8.

Silberg, J., Rutter, M., Meyer J., *et al.* (1996). Genetic and environmental influences on the covariation between hyperactivity and conduct problems in juvenile twins. *Journal of Child Psychology and Psychiatry*, **37**, 803–16.

Thorpe, K., Golding, J., MacGillivray, I., and Greenwood, R. (1991). Comparison of prevalence of depression in mothers of twins and mothers of singletons. *British Medical Journal*, **302**, 875–8.

Werner, E. E., Bierman, J. M., and French, F. E. (1971). *The children of Kauai: a longitudinal study from the prenatal period to age ten.* London, University of Hawaii Press.

Verhulst F. C. and Koot, H. M. (1995). *The epidemiology of child and adolescent psychopathology.* Oxford, Oxford University Press.

4

Promoting our well-being – young views: a study of young people aged 13–19 in Britain

Adrienne Katz

'A strong family background really helps me to have the confidence to do this. They're behind me every step I take.'

'My parents work incredibly hard. I don't load my own problems on to them at the end of the day. We are hardly together enough anyway, and if we are I feel it would upset them.'

'I see these Dads and sons – the father can't see that his son is in trouble, he can't cope with it.'

'You're in your room like, and desperate – and he's reading the paper downstairs. He has no idea about your life.'

'On a very large scale a lot of boys who appear totally OK, inside are falling apart. The difficulty arises in trying to help them. There are stereotypes, social things expected of them.'

This chapter is in two parts. The first part gives an overview of research involving children and the expression of their views. The second part reports on some key findings from two national studies that have been undertaken by *Young Voice*, a national charity which aims to listen and respond to young people, together with Ann Buchanan and her associates at Oxford.

Background: the voice of the child in research

Since the 1989 UN Convention on the Rights of the Child, bringing with it the child's right to be heard and to receive information on the decisions that affect his/her life (Clauses 12–17), it is perhaps not surprising that, over the last ten years, there has been a huge growth in research eliciting children's views on a wide range of subjects.

At much the same time as the growth of the Children's Rights movement have come sociological insights that children are social actors rather than passive recipients of social processes (Prout 1998). This international trend towards studying children as social actors has shifted the research questions and encouraged a greater focus on how children see and act upon their world. For example, in the recent Economic Social Research Council programme on children aged 5–16, some of the research questions were: do children have a particular view and experience of their social, organisational, material, and environmental circumstances – and if so, what is this view? How can they been seen as agents influencing as well as being influenced by social relations, interpreting meanings, and constructing society alongside other actors? How do their own experiences and responses to their social circumstances operate in relation to policies directed toward them? What are the consequences of dividing children's lives between their different contexts rather than seeing them holistically?

Linked to this are more practical considerations: if we want to promote the well-being of children and young people, we need to know how children perceive their world and which responses might be appropriate. In a fast-changing period, adults cannot make assumptions about how young people are processing their experiences (Caprara and Rutter 1995).

The anxieties involved in such research

It is interesting today to read the early concerns about involving children in research. Atwood and Sedighsarvestani, writing in 1979, examined the limitations, and ethical and social issues involved when using children as research subjects. The paper cautioned that the nature of tasks and instrumentation must be especially geared to children; the peculiarities of language development and differential perceptual skills had also to be considered. Researchers were warned not to interpret responses from an adult of point of view. Kayser (1974) and Budd *et al.* (1981) warned that response bias in survey research was especially pronounced among children. Caution was also advised in depending too much on children's reports about their parents' activities (Kayser 1974). Budd *et al.* (1981) noted that, depending on how questions were asked, answers varied dramatically. Ferguson (1978) raised issues about the child's right to make a choice about participation in research. She argued that since the child is considered to be a person with the right of self-determination, three principles are assumed: (1) the child is not the chattel of his/her parents; (2) each individual has the right to make an informed and uncoerced choice; and (3) generation and discovery of knowledge and truth is considered in itself desirable. She suggested that at different age groups different conditions about informed consent should apply, and that children should be given explanations consonant with their level of understanding. Waksler (1986), although welcoming the sociological study of children, noted that the major disadvantage to this approach is that adults, scientists included, commonly reject children's ideas. Two fundamental adult biases that distort data on children were considered. First that children are unfinished in process and secondly that children are routinely wrong, in error, and don't understand. She suggested that suspending these biases enables children to be studied from their own perspective and allows insights into their abilities, knowledge, and ways of being in the world.

Many of these anxieties remain today. Neale *et al.* (1998), for example, explore the potentially conflicting ways of conceptualising children: first as agents of their own lives, and second as dependants in need of protection. They examined these issues in relation to research on families' lives and legal proceedings under the private law provisions of the Children Act 1989. In their studies of post-divorce families they found that children, while being dependent on their families and extremely vulnerable, were social and moral agents negotiating their relationships with existing and new kin. Neale *et al.* (1998) questioned why in a legal context, despite legislative principles that accord children rights, children are still construed as dependants whose needs must be determined for them. Earlier Goodman (1984) highlighted the dilemma. Although children have been testifying in courts of law for centuries, there has always been some concern about the value of their statements. Indeed, early studies on child witnesses by child psychologists supported the stereotype that children were 'the most dangerous of all witnesses'. Goodman (1984) concluded that recent studies have challenged this over-simplified view and suggested that children are not always more suggestible than adults. Amato and Ochiltree (1987) are among the more recent scientists exploring the quality of data when interviewing children. In a study in Australia, they found that agreement between parents and children on ten relatively objective family characteristics was generally high, particularly with older children. Even so, the quality of data for primary school children was high in absolute terms.

Young people's views have been elicited through nationally representative surveys such as the Youth Cohort Study, a young persons' questionnaire linked to the British Household Panel Study (Papasolomontos and Christie 1998); and the 2020 Vision Programme Report, *Speaking Up – Speaking Out!*, for The Industrial Society 1997, in which focus groups, surveys, and mobile survey units were used to elicit responses from almost 10 000 people aged 12–25.

Longitudinal studies prove valuable in assessing relationships between young people's values and attitudes held at one age, and behaviour at another. Buchanan and Ten Brinke (1997) found young people's attitudes aged 16, in 1974 in the National Child Development Study, were remarkably predictive of adult psychological status in 1991. The West of Scotland Twenty-07 study (Sweeting and West 1995) provides a longitudinal study of community health involving 1009 fifteen year olds interviewed at baseline and followed up at 16, 18, 21 and 23 years of age. Such studies have brought a wealth of knowledge and insights for educationalists, health providers, social policy analysts, and others.

As the longitudinal studies continue, further opportunities will arise to assess the relationships between young people's attitudes held at one age and later behaviour (e.g. Buchanan and Ten Brinke 1997). Zinnecker (1999), in an overview of Voice of the Child and Children's Rights research in Europe, notes that the main research topics have been children's poverty; homelessness and the life of street kids; schooling; stress and learning; the role of the peer society; children's constructions of their life course; and justice between generations.

At the other end of the scale, smaller studies on children's perceptions on issues immediately relevant to their lives have also been informative. For example Wenger and Copeland (1994) undertook a study of the coping strategies of low income black children; D'Auria, *et al.* (1997) undertook a small qualitative study on children's perceptions of growing up with cystic fibrosis.

At the community level children's views have also informed the new community policies. Polivka *et al.* (1998) involved 379 inner-city elementary youths in assessing their community. They used a qualitative word association format with the older children, asking them to identify areas of the neighbourhood as 'dirty', 'safe', 'quiet', or 'dangerous'. In Northern Ireland children's perceptions of negative events, using a 25-item self-report measure, were monitored over a 10-year period ending 1994 (Muldoon *et al.* 1998). This found that children's perceptions of stressful and non-stressful events remained relatively constant over time. Those children who lived in working class families, regardless of their religious group, were exposed to greater levels of stress.

Topical media stories have also been the subject of study and their impact on children and young people's values have been researched. Kelley *et al.* (1999) explored the perceptions and reactions of school-age children to information surrounding President Clinton's situation. Data was collected during the 2-week period following publication of the 1998 Starr Report using semi-structured and open questions. Major themes that came from the children were the consequences of lying, getting caught, infidelity and role modelling. They found that parents were often unaware of their children's depth of knowledge and understanding.

With the new studies have come increasingly sophisticated methodologies to plumb the deep recesses of younger and younger children's worlds. Amongst these are surveys, ethnographic approaches, and action research. Focus groups, workbooks and, carton figures have also proved useful. Each approach has to be tailored to the child, his/her age, and the situation and topic under research. All approaches have their strengths but also their limitations. The concerns about the ethical responsibilities of researching with young children remain. Some may be concerned by Finkelhor's (1998) approach to 2000 10- and 11-year-olds, which used a national telephone survey for accessing sensitive kinds of victimisation such as sexual abuse. Surprisingly, he found few difficulties accessing the sample, although parents were slightly more likely to bar the younger respondents, but he found that the young respondents gave important information.

A further concern, as found in an earlier study of children being looked after in state care (Buchanan *et al.* 1993) is that children's responses differ marginally by the contexts and methods used. Confidentiality and trust is important if children are to feel safe to share their deeper concerns. In the Youth Cohort Study, to overcome these concerns young people were given a pre-recorded tape of questions on a walkman and had to record their responses in an answer booklet. This overcame three practical and methodological problems associated with inter-viewing young people within a household environment. It was cost-effective as the questionnaire for the young people was administered at the same time as face-to face interviews were carried out with other adult members of the household; it ensured that the young person felt able to respond honestly and without fear of being overheard by other family members; and it ensured privacy and helped overcome possible literacy problems (Smith 1996).

Young Voice, in the study described below, has been con-cerned to protect the child's right to privacy, and choice of whether or not to participate. Equally, respondents were seen as having an entitlement to know what the research found, and to have that made available to them in accessible form.

This study

In this study, some 4500 young people from all over Great Britain highlighted their experiences of growing up in 1990s Britain. It explored their concerns and problems, their hopes and beliefs on a wide range of issues. By comparing a group of young people who reported high levels of confidence, optimism, and self motivation – the *Can-do* group, with those who were lacking in these attributes – the *Low Can-do* group, further clues emerge on how to promote young people's well-being.

The studies were based on two questionnaires published in *The Express* newspaper. Further copies were delivered to a comparative group of schools and youth clubs. The questionnaires were devised in consultation with a range of children's agencies including Childline, Brook Advisory Centres, The Sex Education Forum at the National Children's Bureau, Young Minds, and researchers at Oxford. Youth workers, teachers, and parents' groups also contributed ideas.

The survey of girls took place on 1 September 1996 and the survey of boys on 1 March 1998. Questionnaires were anonymous with a freepost envelope provided. Three weeks were allowed for their return. Almost 4500 young people took part: 3050 young women and 1400 young men, aged 13–19 years.

Accompanying the quantitative data were a series of interviews. These aimed to hear the views of a range of 50 young men and 50 young women. They came from various parts of the country with very different experiences and backgrounds.

As we have seen, accessing information from young people presents many challenges. An ethical requirement is that children and young people have to choose to participate; young people may be inhibited in what they say when they answer in a school setting; they may be reluctant to share their deepest thoughts with an interviewer. Confidentiality must be demonstrably protected. In the boys' study, possible newspaper-readership response bias was checked with a comparison group from schools and youth clubs. The schools group were marginally younger, otherwise there were very few significant differences in the overall responses given. The newspaper route offered the young people complete anonymity and was an economical route for us to access their inner world – the views and attitudes that may inform their behaviour. With these limitations, this study therefore can only add another piece to the jigsaw of information growing up from numerous other studies using different groups of young people and different methodologies.

Analyses

The initial data analyses were undertaken by market research agencies before being transferred to Oxford for more detailed work. A key question in the secondary analyses was: how did young people with high levels of psychological well-being differ from those at the other end of the spectrum? To answer this question a group of 'Can-do' young people were derived from the dataset.

Further sub-groups were also derived. These identified young people who were depressed and/or suicidal; alienated from school; and in trouble with the police. Some of these findings are presented here. Results are presented as percentages of the total number of each derived group. Chi-square was used to test significance between the groups.

Key findings

A Can-do attitude was strongly associated with less likelihood of a young person feeling *depressed or suicidal* (2% Can-do vs. 31% Low Can-do); less likelihood of their being *anti-school* (4% vs. 43%) and less likelihood of them being *in trouble with the police* (14% vs. 37%). Strikingly, 11% of the Low Can-do boys fell into all three of these categories and 7% fell into two. A key finding, as illustrated in the following Venn Diagrams, is that 83% of the

Table 4.1 Deriving the 'Can-do' sample

	Can-do answer	Low Can-do answer
Do you feel happy and confident about yourself? *and*	Often	Sometimes, hardly ever
There are exciting opportunities for me *and either*	Agree	Disagree
I just get on with my work *or*	Always	Partly true/not true
I set myself high standards	Always	Sometimes/never

334 boys (25% of the sample) were categorised as Can-do.
638 girls (21% of the sample) were categorised as Can-do.
167 boys (13% of the sample) were categorised as Low Can-do.
241 girls (8% of the sample) were categorised as Low Can-do.

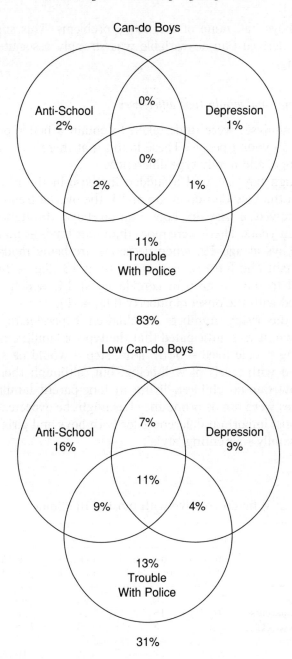

Fig. 4.1 Venn diagrams of the 334 Can-do boys and the 167 Low Can-do boys.

Can-do boys had none of the above problems. This suggested that the derived Can-do variable was strongly associated with well-being.

Gender, age, and family-type differences

Further analyses were undertaken to obtain a better profile of the Can-do young people. These found that there were marked gender, age, and family-type differences.

Although boys showed a sudden increase in the number of people in the Low Can-do group at 14, the overall trend among them showed a rise in Low Can-do boys throughout the adolescent years. There were more than four times as many Low Can-do boys at age 19, when decisions are being made about employment and futures, as there were at 13 (Fig. 4.2a). Girls appeared to have a drop in confidence at 14, which may be associated with the onset of puberty (Fig. 4.2b).

With the rising numbers of children experiencing family breakdown, it was anticipated that the type of families in which the young people lived – birth, lone, step – would be strongly associated with levels of well-being: but, although there were more Low Can-do children living in lone-parent families, the differences were not as pronounced as might be expected.

The most important differences for both boys and girls related to their family's parenting 'style'.

Table 4.2 Who do you live with most of the time?

	Girls		Boys	
	Can-Do % (n = 638)	Low Can-do % (n = 241)	Can-Do % (n = 334)	Low Can-do % (n = 167)
My parents	79	70	78	65
One of my parents	10	15	14	20
Parent and a step family	9	8	3	5
Other	2	7	5	10
Total	100	100	100	100

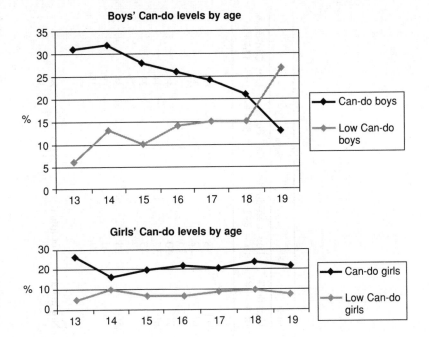

Fig. 4.2 Age and gender differences.

Parenting style

Positive parenting

Can-do children were associated with parents employing a positive parenting style, that is those who:

- Listened to problems and views
- Encouraged initiative
- Were not overly controlling
- Treated everyone in the family equally/fairly
- Provided strict but fair rules (more popular among boys than girls)
- Didn't insist that sons 'acted like a man' or dealt with problems alone
- Offered guidance about life
- Were loving
- Got the young people's respect

Table 4.3 Parenting and Family matters

	Girls		Boys	
	Can-do % (n = 638)	Low Can-do % (n = 241+)	Can-do % (n = 334+)	Low Can-do % (n = 167+)
Parenting style				
My parents are loving – 'yes'	94	68	97	64
My parents listen to my problems and views – 'yes'	66	32	75	27
My parents talk about things that concern me – 'daily'	31	13	23	7
My parents like me to make my own decisions – 'yes'	70	40	70	44
My parents are helpful – 'yes'	69	37	83	44
My parents offer guidance – 'yes'	50	25	59	21
My parents lay down the right rules – 'yes'			71	35
My parents treat everyone in the family alike – 'yes'	50	25	72	38
They take no notice of me – 'agree'	8	10	10	19
My parents try to control everything I do – 'yes'	6	19	7	25
Father/son relationship				
Is your dad living with you – 'yes'	Not asked	Not asked	81	71
Living elsewhere, but I see him – 'yes'			20	32
Another man acts as your father – 'yes'				

Does your father:				
spend time with you?	8	Not asked	Not asked	21
hug you? – 'yes'	81	Not asked	Not asked	35
show an interest in your schoolwork? – 'yes'	29	Not asked	Not asked	10
talk through your worries with you? – 'yes'	79	Not asked	Not asked	35
believe you should fight your own battles? – 'yes'	42	Not asked	Not asked	12
talk to you about relationships? – 'yes'	34	Not asked	Not asked	44
	26	Not asked	Not asked	3
Do you see yourself as a father – NO	6	Not asked	Not asked	23
Family 'togetherness'				
How often do you usually do things together?				
Watch TV/video – 'daily'	62	72	56	41
Eat a meal together – 'daily'	77	31	20	49
Visit friends and relatives – 'weekly'	41	22	10	19
Walk or play sport – 'weekly'	39	Not asked	Not asked	13
Arguing				
My parents fight a lot with each other – 'yes'	5	Not asked	Not asked	17
How often do you argue with your parents – 'daily'	13	Not asked	21	27
Attitude to parents				
Do you plan to look after your children as you have been – 'yes'	55	42	20	19

The lives of the Can-do group appeared to be dramatically different from those who were Low Can-do. Boys in this group were, for example, more than six times as likely to take an illegal drug when very distressed. They were poor at communicating and seemed 'cut off' and isolated sometimes from relationships and generally from news, guidance, and information. They were two and a half times more likely to have been in trouble with the police and eight times more likely to be deeply anti-school.

Emotional support

A marked difference between boys and girls was apparent when asked to whom they would turn for emotional support. Girls, as a group, were far more likely than boys to turn to friends because this involved no loss of face. Of girls, 84% would turn to a friend while only 48% of boys would do so.

A girl explains: 'If you're in the habit of moaning to a friend about your acne, then it's easy to tell her something worse has happened to you.' But a typical male remark was: 'I wouldn't talk to a friend about a problem – most boys wouldn't. He's a mate, for having a laugh and that.' Or 'If you tell a mate he might tell others and they'll think you're pathetic.'

Mothers, however, were usually the main source of support for boys and girls, but the extent to which they were used differed by gender. Whereas 72% of *all* girls would turn to their mother when they needed help, only 58% of boys would do so despite the fact that they listed their mothers as the most fre-quently used source. The differences between the Can-do and Low Can-do groups were more marked than gender differences: over 75% of Can-do boys and girls indicated that they turn to their mothers for emotional support compared to only 44% of Low Can-do boys and 60% of Low Can-do girls. In addition Can-do girls were far more likely than their Low Can-do counterparts to put their mother as their first choice. Low Can-do girls were more likely to say they turn to friends in the first instance.

Fathers (or father figures – this study did not differentiate between the two) were rarely a prime source of emotional sup-port for boys. Although 61% of Can-do boys said they did some-times turn to Dad, only 14% named him as the prime source.

Only 23% of Low Can-do boys named a father as a source of comfort at all. These boys were far more likely to turn to friends or teachers for help. Earlier work by Buchanan and Ten Brinke (1997) suggests that who you turn to in times of need indicates an expectation that that person is both *willing* and *able* to give the necessary support. In this situation it is possible that the Low Can-do boys were making a judgement that their father was not able (maybe he did not live with them) or not willing to help. Fathers who were involved with their children, however, proved to be important.

Father or 'father' figure involvement

In an analysis of family structure and substance abuse risk, CASA in the US (Centre on Addiction and Substance Abuse 1999) found that children living in two-parent families who have a fair or poor relationship with their father are at 68% higher risk of smoking, drinking, and using drugs compared with all teens living in a two-parent household, while children growing up in a home headed by a single mother, who have an excellent relationship with her are at 62% lower risk of abusing substances than those in a two-parent family with a fair or poor relationship with their father. Where the father is pro-active and caring, very good outcomes are noted. 'The safest teens are those . . . who have a positive relationship with both parents, go to both parents equally when they have decisions to make.'

In this study, girls who reported a supportive father were more likely to be in the Can-do group. His input appeared to give a disproportionate boost to a girl's confidence and self belief.

For boys, the role of father or 'father-figure' was strongly associated with emotional well-being. Fathers of Can-do boys were more than twice as likely to spend time with their sons and twice as likely to take an interest in their school work. The Can-do boys were three times as likely to be hugged by their dads as Low Can-do boys.

More than 70% of all boys studied lived with their fathers. One in five of the Can-do boys had a dad who lived elsewhere whom they saw regularly, but amongst the Low Can-do boys twice as many had another man acting as a father and twice as many had an absent father.

Some fathers, according to the young men, were physically present while emotionally absent or unavailable to their sons.

Because this study did not differentiate between fathers and father-figures, the quantitative findings are a little ambivalent. Some father-figures may be grandfathers, uncles, or friends. In the interviews with young people, it was apparent that several absent fathers maintained a good relationship with their sons. The relationship between the parents, however, has its own dynamic. Having a poor relationship with a father or fighting parents might be worse than not having any relationship at all with a father. Watching parents argue at age 7, for example, has been found to have a significant relationship with arguing with your parents at age 16 and with your partner at age 33 (Buchanan and Ten Brinke 1997).

Further analyses on a derived variable for high and low levels of father involvement (father spends time with me; listens to my

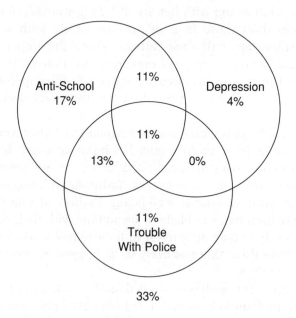

Fig. 4.3 Low father involvement.

concerns and worries; takes an interest in my school work), found that, among boys, low father involvement showed strong relationships with alienation from school, depression and suicide, and police involvement.

Family togetherness

'Family togetherness' has been found to play an important part as young as age seven in protecting against depression in later life (Buchanan and Ten Brinke 1998), and in protecting against substance misuse (Centre on Addiction and Substance Abuse 1999). In the West of Scotland Study (Sweeting and West 1995), children in families that did things together were protected from a range of social ills.

In this study, too, aspects of family togetherness were strongly associated with emotional well-being. Further analyses of a 'family togetherness'-derived variable (families who eat a meal together 'daily'; visit friends and relatives 'weekly'; walk or play sport 'weekly') found that high levels of family togetherness were protective against depression and school disaffection. Three quarters of the boys with high levels of family togetherness did not become depressed or disaffected or get into trouble with the police.

At the other end of the scale, as illustrated in Fig. 4.4, 32% of those boys with low family togetherness fell into the disaffected category; 35% had been in trouble with the police and 24% were depressed; 12% were both anti-school and in trouble with the police. Only 39% of those with low family togetherness remained outside any of these three categories.

Schools

There is an attitude among some boys that learning is uncool. There is also a feeling in society that scientists, teachers and doctors are not valued. It affects boys' attitudes to education. (Boy of 17)

Although it has long been known that the social context and 'ethos' of the school can play a key role in a child's levels of

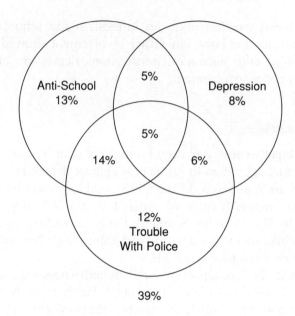

Fig. 4.4 Low family togetherness.

achievement and emotional well-being (Rutter *et al.* 1979; Olweus 1993), in recent years the views of young people, particularly around bullying, have added fuel to this fire.

In this study a strong relationship was seen between levels of Can-do attitude and school issues. The high self-esteem boys were more likely to be in a school with an anti-bullying policy and a school with a policy that they believed was 'working'. Bullying and violence were the daily fare of too many young people. Two-thirds of Low Can-do boys whose school *had* an anti-bullying policy, did *not* think it was working.

Self-esteem took a knock from other children but young people also complained that they were sometimes made to feel stupid by their teachers. More than a quarter of Low Can-do boys said '*You are made to feel stupid if you make a mistake.*' Injured pride and anger at being made to seem a fool in front of peers appeared to act as a blocker to learning and co-operation. '*You gotta get respect.*' (Boy of 18)

Table 4.4 School experience

School	Girls		Boys	
	Can-do % (n = 638+)	Low Can-do % (n = 241+)	Can-do % (n = 334+)	Low Can-do % (n = 167+)
Views about school and teachers				
School				
Girls: I do not like it – 'not true at all'. Boys: It is a waste of time – 'not true'	88	46	82	39
I like my teachers and enjoy school – 'very true'	48	10	47	12
Teachers don't know me as a person – 'very true'.	Not asked	Not asked	20	51
You are made to feel stupid if you don't understand – 'very true'	Not asked	Not asked	10	27
Have you had good career advice? – 'yes', 'always'	64	36	74	35
School ethos and bullying				
Bullying in school – Have you been:				
physically attacked? – 'a little or a lot'	13	25	29	53
been threatened with violence? – 'a little or a lot'	20	34	35	58
Does your school have an anti-bullying policy? – 'yes'	54	34	72	38
Do you think the anti-bullying policy is working – 'no'	52	75	38	66
Is bullying affecting your life – 'a lot or a bit'	Not asked	Not asked	10	27
Have you ever bullied someone? – 'a lot or a little'	21	32	30	38

Meeting goals

Girls were more likely to feel they would achieve their goals, yet more boys than girls are certain about what they want to do in the future. Low Can-do young people are less able to visualise themselves with a job and a family or do not necessarily want this.

Table 4.5 Meeting goals

	Girls		Boys	
	Can-do % (*n* = 638)	Low Can-do % (*n* = 241)	Can-do % (*n* = 334)	Low Can-do % (*n* = 167)
I want a job and a family and I'll cope – 'Yes'	81	62	93	67

Experience of violence

Low Can-do girls and boys were significantly more likely to say they had experienced being hit or beaten and an adult making violent threats, as shown in Table 4.6. They were also more likely to say they were bullied outside school. Among those who were depressed or suicidal, the experience of violence from adults was one of the most significant findings.

Table 4.6 Boys' experience of violence

	Not depressed % (*n* = 1192)	Depressed % (*n* = 152)	Not suicidal % (*n* = 817)	Suicidal % (*n* = 40)
Have you experienced an adult using violence against you? – 'Yes, a little/a lot'	20	43	16	69

The more worrying groups

Boys alienated from school

When a subgroup of 227 boys who were anti-school was derived from the data, it was found that they were more likely than other boys to believe:

'It's harder for men these days' (68% vs. 56%)

'It was easier when roles for men and women were clearly separate' (57% vs. 42%), and

'Boys are expected to match up to one ideal of maleness' (44% vs. 32%)

This evidence of a backlash emphasises other findings from this study suggesting that boys with low self-esteem need help to come to terms with social change and that we should pay attention to their feelings of resentment. They tended to make the much publicised academic success of girls an excuse for their own poor performance. The logic of this was that 'doing well at school is a girly thing and I don't want to appear girly', so the *mega macho thing is to muck about.*' They gain more admiration from peers if they make trouble than if they are seen as stupid. Being thought of as girlish was anathema and therefore behaviour had to become more 'laddish' to compensate and differentiate males from females. Homophobic bullying was reported widely in interviews.

Boys have to be hard, if they're not like that they're not liked by other men. The hard image comes through family – you try to follow them. Boys try not to look small, even if they feel small. (Boy of 14)

The disaffected subgroup echoed many trends found among Low Can-do boys but in addition the lack of parental interest in their school lives was clear. Family life for the disaffected boys was marked by a harsher regime: they were twice as likely to argue daily with parents as other boys, less likely to eat together, and over half 'rarely or never' visit friends and relatives as a family. All family togetherness activities, ranging from TV watching to playing a sport, took place less often in their lives. Only 35% of disaffected boys said 'my parents listen to my problems and views' vs. 61% of all other boys. Few of their fathers took an interest in schoolwork (37% vs. 66%) or talked through worries with them (15% vs. 30%).

The depressed and suicidal

More than one in ten Low Can–do boys had attempted suicide. Although levels of depression were similar among both girls and boys, for the latter there were significant barriers to getting help. Cultural assumptions about how boys and men behave, weaker support networks, and a lack of communication skills were among the barriers this study found. For many boys, as shown above, their fathers did not appear to be available for them. Peer group behaviour among young men was a powerful force inhibiting any self-revelation.

Antisocial behaviour in boys was demonstrably linked to suicidal behaviour. Twenty per cent of the depressed and 50% of the suicidal boys in this study said they had been in trouble with the police. Recent research (Buchanan and Ten Brinke 1998) has highlighted that young men with antisocial behaviour, who may have had an externalising behaviour disorder from a young age, are at risk of depression in late adolescence and early adulthood. A rise in depressive disorder amongst young people and its onset at an earlier age, and an increase in substance misuse have been put forward as explanations for the 60% increase in suicidal behavioural in the under-25s over the period 1981–91 (Samaritans 1999).

Use of drugs

Both girls' and boys' surveys revealed that young people believe that parents do not give enough clear and useful information about drugs. In addition, 85% of boys were concerned that drug use was spreading to younger boys; 60% were worried about the effects of drugs on those around them and 40% were worried about the effects on themselves. Low self-esteem boys were significantly less worried about the effects on themselves, but ranked drugs highly as a cause of stress. (They may live with a drug user or be surrounded by a culture of drug misuse.) Girls who said they had tried drugs gave several reasons for doing so. The most common reason was '*to see what it's like*', but 33% did so '*because of depression or tension*'. Boys in the suicidal subgroup were ten times more likely than non-suicidal boys to say they take a drug when worried or upset. Low Can-do boys' spending patterns on drugs, alcohol, and cigarettes vary in a revealing way from those of Can-do boys, as shown in Fig. 4.5.

Sex and relationships education

Girls were unequivocal in asking for more information on a range of health and sex education subjects. Eighty-eight per cent wanted more information on '*where to get help*'. They highlight the poor levels of information provided by parents and, very often, schools, in a population with the highest teenage pregnancy rate in Europe.

Typically, fewer boys admit they need more information and they argue that what has been offered at school is not relevant for them, but too girl-orientated. They report that parents seldom give boys guidance on relationships and sex education with as few as 4% saying they got this from their father. Boys from the depressed/suicidal subgroup were significantly more worried about their lack of knowledge about sex and relationships. Some 75% of them wanted more on '*relationships and emotional feelings*', 61% on '*where to get help*', and 60% on '*Sexuality. Am I different?*'

Information and guidance is needed to counter myths and can alleviate the worry experienced by large numbers of adolescents. The failure of adults to give adequate guidance was evident in personal stories and in statistics. It was not mechanical informa-

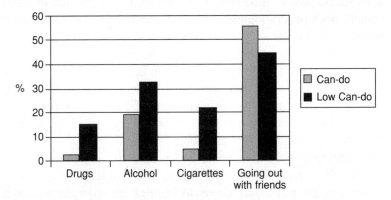

Fig. 4.5 What do you spend your money on? Boys.

tion they felt the lack of, but information on the intangible side of human relationships. It would be helpful for parents and educators to know that over one-third of Can-do boys said they would like more information on *'relationships and emotional feelings'*. Almost one third of Low Can-do boys want more information on *'Sexuality. Am I different?'*

Conclusion

Each study is like a piece of jigsaw. It increases our under-standing of the big picture by adding to the findings from other studies. It is interesting that findings about parenting and family style in this study echo those from other studies. For example Sweeting *et al.* (1998) in the West of Scotland Study found that different outcomes for young people were associated with different aspects of family life, the most constant relationships occurring with respect to time spent in family activities. The majority of the relationships remained after accounting for material deprivation and were the same for males and females. In an earlier study they examined three dimensions of family life: family structure, culture, and conflict, on health outcomes in 1009 young people between the ages of 15 and 18. Despite a strong association between family structure and material depri-vation, respondents with different family structures were largely undifferentiated in terms of health. By contrast, aspects of family functioning were independently associated with lower self-esteem, poor psychological well-being, and, amongst girls, more physical symptoms.

Similarly, in a study using data from the National Child Development Study (Buchanan and Ten Brinke 1997; Buchanan and Ten Brinke 1998) there were also indications that what goes on within the family – involvement of father, outings with mother, lack of family conflict – is positively linked to positive outcomes for children in adulthood.

As young people help us to break into the private world of family life, a clearer vision emerges of what really matters to young people and what needs to change in order to promote their well-being.

References

Amato, P. R. and Ochiltree, G. (1987). Interviewing children about their families: a note on data quality. *Journal of Marriage and the Family*, **49**(3), 669–75.

Atwood, M. E. and Sedighsarvestani, R. (1979). *Children as experimental research subjects in sociology*. Association Paper. North Central Sociological Association, University of Akron, OH, USA.

Buchanan, A. (1995). Young people's views on being looked after in out-of-home-care under the Children Act 1989. *Children and Youth Services Review*, **17**(5–6), 681–96.

Buchanan, A., Wheal, A., Walder, A., Macdonald, S. and Coker, R. (1993). *Answering back: Report by young people on the Children Act, 1989*. Southampton CEDR, University of Southampton.

Buchanan, A and Ten Brinke, J-A. (1997). *What happened when they were grown up? Outcomes from parenting experiences*. York, Joseph Rowntree Foundation /York Publishing.

Buchanan, A. and Ten Brinke, J-A. (1998). *Recovery from emotional and behavioural problems*. Report to NHS Executive Anglia and Oxford.

Budd, E. C., Sigelman, C. K., and Sigelman, L. (1981). Exploring the outer limits of response bias. *Sociological Focus*, **14**(4), 297–307.

Caprara, G. V. and Rutter, M. (1995). Individual development and social change. In M. Rutter and D. J. Smith (eds.), *Psychosocial disorders in young people*. Chichester, Wiley.

Centre on Addiction and Substance Abuse (1999). *The fifth annual CASA national survey of American attitudes on substance abuse in teens and their parents*. Columbia University, New York, Centre on Addiction and Substance Abuse.

D'Auria, J. P., Christian, N. J., and Richardson, L. F. (1997). Through the looking glass: children's perceptions of growing up with cystic fibrosis. *Canadian Journal of Nursing Research*, **29**(4), 99–112.

Ferguson, L. R. (1978). Freedom of children to make choices regarding participation in research: a statement. *Journal of Social Issues*, **34**(4), 114–21.

Finkelhor, D. (1998). A comparison of responses of preadolescents and adolescents in a national victimization survey. *Journal of Interpersonal Violence*, **13**(3), 362–83.

Goodman, G. A. (1984). Children's testimony in historical perspective. *Journal of Social Issues*, **40**(2), 9–31.

The Industrial Society (1997). *Speaking up - speaking out! The 20/20 vision programme research report*. London, The Industrial Society.

Kayser, B. D. (1974). Response bias in children's reports of parental status characteristics. *Sociological Focus*, **7**(2), 61–76.

Kelley, B. R., Beauchesne, M. A., Babington, L. M., *et al.* (1999). The President Clinton crisis and the Starr report: children's perceptions and parents' awareness. *Journal of Pediatric Health Care,* **13**(4), 166–72.

Muldoon, O. T., Trew, K., and McWhirter, L. (1998). Children's perceptions of negative events in Northern Ireland: a ten-year study. *European Child and Adolescent Psychiatry,* **7**(1), 36–41.

Neale, B. and Smart, C. (1998). *Agents or dependants? Struggling to listen to children in family research and family law.* Working Paper no. 3, Centre for Research on Family, Kinship and Childhood, University of Leeds.

Olweus, D. (1993). *Bullying in school: what we know and what we can do.* Oxford, Blackwell.

Papasolomontos, C. and Christie, T. (1998). Using national surveys: a review of secondary analyses with special reference to education. *Educational Research,* **40**(3), 295–310.

Polivka, B. J., Lovell, M., and Smith, B. A. (1998). A qualitative assessment of inner city elementary school children's perceptions of their neighborhood. *Public Health Nursing,* **15**(3), 171–9.

Prout, A. (1998). *Studying children as social actors: a programme of research in the United Kingdom.* Association Paper. American Sociological Association.

Rutter, M., Maughan, B., Mortimore, P., and Ouston, J. (1979). *Fifteen thousand hours: secondary schools and their effects on children.* London, Open Books.

The Samaritans (1999). *Listen up – responding to people in crisis.* London, The Samaritans.

Smith, R. (1996). Capturing sensitive data from young people in a household setting. *Journal of the Market Research Society,* **38**(2), 177–83.

Sweeting, H. and West, P. (1995). Family life and health in adolescence: a role for culture in the health inequalities debate? *Social Science and Medicine,* **40**(2), 163–75.

Sweeting, H., West, P., and Richards, M. (1998). Teenage family life, lifestyles and life changes: associations with family structure, conflict with parents and joint family activity. *International Journal of Law, Policy and the Family,* **12**(1), 15–46.

United Nations (1989). *The UN convention on the rights of the child, 1989.* New York, United Nations.

Waksler, F. C. (1986). Studying children: phenomenological insights. *Human Studies,* **9**(1), 71–82.

Wenger, R. and Copeland, S. G. (1994). Coping strategies used by black school-age children from low-income families. *Journal of Pediatric Nursing,* **9**(1), 33–40.

Zinnecker, J. F. (1999). *The European voice of children. Children's rights movement, social policy for and with children, and the new childhood research.* Association Paper. American Sociological Association.

5

Parent–child interaction and children's well-being: reducing conduct problems and promoting conscience development

Frances Gardner and Sarah Ward

'The components of mental health include the following capacities:

the ability to develop psychologically, emotionally, intellectually and spiritually; the ability to initiate, develop and sustain mutually satisfying personal relationships; the ability to become aware of others and to empathise with them; the ability to use psychological distress as a developmental process, so that it does not hinder or impair further development.'

Health Advisory Service 1995, *Together we stand*, p. 15

Conduct problems in childhood are clearly detrimental to emotional well-being, in both the short and long term. Children with conduct problems have increased rates of depression, peer problems, and school failure. Longitudinal studies indicate that their long-term outlook is also poor. In adulthood, not only are these children at greater risk of physical and mental illness but they also tend to fare much less well academically, in employment, and in relationships with others (Robins 1991). The WHO defines health in these broad terms, as 'a state of total emotional and physical well-being, not merely the absence of illness'. Similarly, children's well-being, as seen above in the Health Advisory Service's definition of mental health, should be seen as more than merely the absence of emotional and behavioural problems. One way to consider promotion of children's well-being, therefore, is to consider factors that will both prevent the development of antisocial tendencies and also provide them with positive guidelines for behaviour. In order to become fully socialised adults, children must (a) acquire a set of moral principles for guiding their behaviour, even in the absence of external controls; (b) develop sensitivity to the feelings of others; (c) learn to recognise that others may have needs which are different from their own; (d) learn self-control in order to inhibit undesirable behaviour; and finally, (e) acquire a repertoire of prosocial behaviours in order to get along with others. These characteristics can be considered to be indicators of having a 'conscience' which guides behaviour (Kochanska 1993; 1997b). This chapter will consider emotional well-being from two angles, examining how parent–child interaction contributes to the development of conduct problems and conscience in young children.

Definition of children's conduct problems

Conduct problems are known by a number of labels in the literature on younger children, including acting-out, externalising, antisocial, hard-to-manage, or non-compliant behaviour. These terms all refer to an empirically derived cluster of problems, known as Oppositional Defiant Disorder in DSM-IV (American Psychiatric Association 1994), and defined as 'recurrent pattern of negativistic, defiant, hostile behaviour' including tempers, non-compliance, spiteful, angry, and resentful behaviour. These behaviours need to persist for many months, to occur more frequently than in other children of the same age, and to cause impairment in the child's social or school functioning. The term 'Conduct Disorder' in DSM-IV refers to more serious antisocial behaviour usually developing later in childhood and often includes oppositional behaviours plus harmful aggression, destructiveness, theft, and rule-breaking. The term 'conduct problems' is used here to refer to the cluster of difficult behaviours defined above.

Definition of conscience

One of the most important developmental transitions in childhood is the shift from other-control to self-control. Schaffer (1996, p. 248) notes that 'in the course of development, children must learn to assume responsibility for their own behaviour . . . the emergence of the capacity for self regulation is one of the hallmarks of childhood and represents an achievement of great complexity'. Children who achieve this could be said to have a moral 'conscience'. Kochanska (1993) argues that affective, cognitive, behavioural, and motivational processes underlie children's ability to refrain from antisocial behaviours. In particular, affective processes such as guilt or empathy motivate a child to behave morally. However, they must also develop the capacity for self-control in order to refrain from antisocial impulses. Furthermore, a positive emotional relationship with the parent motivates the child to accept their values. Other researchers have emphasised the role of empathy in the internalisation of rules (e.g. Hoffman 1975), the development of prosocial behaviour (Eisenberg and Miller 1987), and the inhibition of antisocial behaviour (Miller and Eisenberg 1988). In a later section, we will examine whether aspects of parent–child interaction promote the internalisation of parental rules, the development of a capacity for self-regulation, and the development of affective processes, particularly empathy.

Why are conduct problems important?

Conduct problems in children are common, persistent, difficult to treat (Kazdin 1993), costly to society, and have a poor prognosis (Robins 1991). Longitudinal studies show that antisocial behaviour originates in the pre-school years, resulting from a combination of difficult early temperamental characteristics (White *et al.* 1990; Bates *et al.* 1991) and dysfunctional family interaction (Patterson *et al.* 1992; Reid 1993; Loeber and Hay 1994; Campbell 1995; Dishion *et al.* 1995). These behaviour patterns show a well-documented developmental progression starting with hard-to-manage pre-schoolers, about 50% of whom go on to have more serious oppositional and conduct disorders in middle childhood (Richman *et al.* 1982; Campbell 1995), followed by delinquency in early adolescence.

The detrimental consequences of this behaviour for the well-being of the individual, family, school, and for society are considerable. Antisocial children are more likely to be rejected and victimised by peers (Schwartz *et al.* 1999), to fail at school, and to truant. Their disruptive behaviour in class often leads to school exclusion. The outlook for adult life is also poor. Both clinic- (Robins 1991) and population-based (Fergusson and Horwood 1998; Fergusson and Lynskey 1998) longitudinal studies have found strong continuities between child and adult disorder. Children with conduct disorders have very high rates of antisocial personality disorder, suicide, other mental illness, and criminality. Those who escape these major problems nevertheless have an increased risk of social difficulties such as divorce and drug abuse. Life opportunities are reduced in terms of more unemployment and fewer qualifications, even after controlling for the effects of social disadvantage (Fergusson and Horwood 1998). Childhood conduct disorder is the strongest predictor of later violence towards a partner, and this holds for both boys and girls (Moffitt and Caspi 1998; Capaldi and Clark 1998). Antisocial boys are more likely to become fathers at an early age, thus increasing the likelihood of transmitting difficulties across generations (Capaldi and Stoolmiller 1999; Loeber, pers. comm.). Rydelius (1988) found that the death rate was higher for antisocial children than the general population, especially for violent death. The fact that conduct problems start young, are stable, and have a clear progression to more serious outcomes makes a strong argument for carrying out early intervention to help prevent later disorder. Although good results have been obtained in trials of parenting interventions with antisocial adolescents (Dishion *et al.* 1996), there is evidence that these problems are more difficult to treat in older children when difficulties become entwined with the child's peer relations, school failure, and petty crime, and the child and his family feel stigmatised, isolated, and hopeless (Webster-Stratton 1998).

Why is the development of conscience important?

The development of conscience is in itself an important goal of socialisation, since it involves moral and empathic awareness and self-control. However, there are two main reasons why conscience development is also important for improving long-term outcomes for children with conduct disorder.

Firstly, researchers have begun to recognise the importance of covert antisocial behaviours, such as lying, stealing, and fire-setting, as well as overt behaviours such as aggression and defiance (Loeber 1990; Frick *et al.* 1993; Loeber *et al.* 1993). Longitudinal studies indicate that the prognosis is worse for children who engage in covert as well as overt antisocial behaviours (Loeber *et al.* 1997). It follows, therefore, that identification of factors which could prevent the development of covert antisocial tendencies would help to improve the prognosis for children with conduct disorder. The influence of parent–child interaction on the development of aggression and defiance has been well-documented (e.g. Patterson 1982; Patterson *et al.* 1992). Less is known about the influence of parent–child interaction on the development of covert antisocial behaviours. However, research suggests that a number of parenting behaviours may promote the development of conscience in young children. It is argued that the development of a moral conscience, including an internalised set of moral standards, underlies children's ability to refrain from behaving antisocially in the absence of external controls. Thus conscience development is likely to be particularly important for preventing an individual from engaging in covert antisocial acts.

Secondly, one of the most serious outcomes for children with conduct disorder is Antisocial Personality Disorder (APD). This is characterized by an extreme lack of conscience, and is defined by DSM-IV (American Psychiatric Association 1994) as 'a pervasive pattern of disregard for and violation of the rights of others' indicated by behaviours such as criminal behaviour, deceitfulness, impulsivity, aggressiveness, recklessness, irresponsibility, and a lack of remorse for harm caused to others. Robins *et al.* (1991) found that 70% of children with severe conduct disorder beginning before age 6 go on to develop APD in adulthood, compared to only 25% of those with mild conduct disorder. This raises questions about how and when the remaining children improve, and which children are most at risk. Factor analytic studies indicate there are two distinct traits characterising individuals with APD: psychopathy/emotional detachment and antisocial behaviour (Frick *et al.* 1994). The combination of antisocial and psychopathic traits is highly predictive of forensic status and of severe and chronic antisocial behaviour (Harpur *et al.* 1989; Hare *et al.* 1991).

Frick *et al.* (1994) argue that the predictors of antisocial behaviour are somewhat different from the predictors of psychopathy/emotional detachment. They found that antisocial behaviour was related to adverse family environment, low SES and low intelligence, whereas emotional detachment was positively related to traits such as narcissism and negatively with anxiety. Furthermore, Patrick *et al.* (1997) found that emotionally detached offenders were less likely to come from socially disadvantaged environments than other offenders. It follows, therefore, that research which focuses solely on the development of antisocial behaviour in children with conduct disorder cannot explain the whole picture regarding antisocial personality disorder. This disorder is poorly understood and extremely costly and hard to treat. A possible solution would be to develop early prevention programmes, but first it is necessary to gain an understanding of its developmental origins and possible causal mechanisms. It is argued, therefore, that it is important to examine conscience development in children with conduct disorder, in order to see if conscience can help predict who will develop more serious antisocial personality disorder in adulthood.

Research methods for assessing parenting style and its contribution to child behaviour

The most thoroughly researched causal factor in the development of conduct problems and conscience is parenting behaviour. There is particularly strong evidence, converging from several different kinds of research design, that parenting style contributes to the development and maintenance of conduct problems. The study of how parenting contributes to conscience development is less well developed, with fewer studies (Kochanska and Aksan 1995 is an exception) using observational methods or more informative longitudinal and experimental designs. We will first outline important features of research measurement and design that attempt to investigate these questions, and then describe some of the studies in more detail.

Systematic observational techniques

The development of systematic observational techniques for assessing parent and child behaviour in their natural context has been essential to the development of this field. These techniques are the only way to assess in fine detail what takes place, moment-by-moment, during an interaction. Understanding interaction on this level has proved very useful for predicting child outcomes and for devising effective interventions (Forehand and McMahon 1981; Patterson 1982; Gardner *et al.* 1999a; Patterson and Forgatch 1995; Gardner 1997). Some of the first detailed observational measures of parent–child interaction in the home were developed by Patterson and colleagues (Reid 1978; Patterson 1982), who paid careful attention to testing the reliability and validity of their measures. Earlier studies of parenting and behaviour problems used interview measures of parenting style (Sears *et al.* 1957; Baumrind 1967), but the validity of these instruments was not well tested against observational and other techniques (Maccoby and Martin 1983). Recently there have been attempts to validate more focused interview measures of parenting against direct observational findings. Some studies have found reasonable convergence (Kochanska *et al.* 1989; Webster-Stratton and Spitzer 1991; Webster-Stratton 1998) and other studies slight (Deater-Deckard *et al.* 1996) or poor convergence (Patterson *et al.* 1992; p. 68) between observational and interview measures. There have not been enough studies to allow us to say which aspects of parenting, if any, can be adequately measured using self-report, and which techniques are most useful. The evidence to date suggests that direct observations are the most useful way of measuring parent–child interaction.

Research designs for examining the causal role of parenting

Correlational designs Many studies have used correlational designs to demonstrate associations between parenting style and child behaviour. These studies are very important in describing systematically how parenting varies across families, and how it relates to child behaviour (Patterson 1982; Gardner 1989, 1994; Campbell 1995; Dumas *et al.* 1995). However, correlational designs are viewed as insufficient for demonstrating that parenting influences problem behaviour, since any associations found may be interpreted in a number of ways (Loeber and Farrington 1994). For instance, correlations may be interpreted as showing that parenting influences child behaviour, but equally the causal direction could be the other way round, or the association due to other factors, for example the influence of a hostile neighbourhood, or genetic factors, which may affect both parenting and child behaviour. Rutter (1994a) takes a more constructive view, pointing to strengths of correlational designs that are not always recognised. He argues that it is essential to establish correlations between variables before deciding which questions to test in costly longitudinal studies. Moreover he suggests that there are circumstances in which correlational designs can be an important part of a series of tests of a causal hypothesis, for example where the opportunity for a 'natural experiment' occurs, and in the testing of competing hypotheses.

Longitudinal designs These have the advantage of being able to show how a risk factor predicts an outcome that is measured later in time, but do not completely get round the problem of interpreting the direction of causality (see Loeber and Farrington 1994; Rutter 1994a for a fuller discussion of strengths and limitations). A number of longitudinal observational studies have shown that parenting influences later conduct problems, whilst controlling for the powerful predictive effects of earlier levels of conduct problems (e.g. Zahn-Waxler *et al.* 1990; Shaw *et al.* 1994b; Shaw *et al.* 1998; Gardner *et al.* 1999a,b).

Intervention and experimental designs These are powerful designs for establishing causes, but suffer from the drawback that the effects of contrived interventions may tell us more about the possible impact of parenting in the context of a therapeutic intervention than about its naturally occurring effects. Bryant (1985) and Loeber and Farrington (1994) suggest that a solution may be to combine experimental intervention with naturalistic longitudinal studies, in order to bring together the advantages of both. These approaches have not been applied to the study of conscience. However, many studies of conduct problems have employed one of these designs, providing evidence for the causal role of parenting style, but few studies have combined the two approaches. There have been numerous controlled trials of parenting interventions which attempt to change parents' style of dealing with difficult behaviour, and show predicted improvements in child behaviour (Patterson 1982; Webster-Stratton *et al.* 1989; Webster-Stratton 1994; 1998; Cunningham *et al.* 1995; Tremblay *et al.* 1995; Sanders *et al.* in press; for reviews see Serketich and Dumas 1996; Barlow 1998; Taylor and Biglan 1998). Some studies show that changes in parent behaviour per se are crucial predictors of child outcome (e.g. Patterson and Forgatch 1995), providing further evidence for the causal role of parenting variables. There have also been some examples of more tightly controlled experimental interventions which manipulate only one or two specified aspects of parent behaviour, thus allowing more precise identification of the effects of particular parenting variables on child behaviour. For example Forgatch (1991), Dishion *et al.* (1992), Patterson *et al.* (1992), and Reid *et al.* (1994) have shown that teaching more consistent discipline strategies led to decreases in antisocial behaviour.

Behaviour genetic studies using twin and adoption designs   These are important because they have the power both to show how weak or strong is the genetic influence on behaviour, and to tell us more about the extent and nature of environmental influences, such as parenting (Plomin 1994), and whether these influences are shared between sibs or unique to that child. For example, an adoption study by Deater-Deckard and Plomin (in press), and large twin studies (Eaves *et al.* 1997; Gjone and Stevenson 1997) found a moderate influence of both genetic and shared environmental factors on conduct problems. However, these and other studies have mainly used self-report measures of behaviour (e.g. Simonoff *et al.* 1995) and have found that the relative contribution of these factors varied, sometimes a great deal, depending on the sample, the informant, and the type of measure used (Rutter *et al.* 1999). There have been fewer studies of genetic influences on observed behaviour, which is noteworthy, since one twin study found no genetic effects on observed aggression (Plomin *et al.* 1990). This stands in contrast to many questionnaire studies which find large genetic effects on aggression. Other studies suggest the importance of environmental influences that are not shared by the twins or sibs, but are unique to individuals (Plomin 1994). These findings raise interesting questions about the extent to which parents direct their behaviour selectively to different children in the family. This could result from factors such as child temperamental differences (non-genetic), or variations in parental mental state or attitudes affecting one child and not the other at an important developmental stage. These factors would interact with parenting styles to produce individual child outcomes. Behaviour genetic designs also offer the exciting possibility of using observational methods to examine genetic and environmental sources of influence on parenting and child behaviour, and on the associations between parent and child behaviour.

Parenting and conduct problems

Social factors and parenting

As well as parenting, wider social factors have an influence on conduct problems. Rutter's (1978) epidemiological studies found a set of 'family adversity' factors, including maternal depression, marital discord, overcrowding, low social class, and paternal antisocial behaviour, that were strongly related to conduct disorder in middle childhood. These findings have been replicated in later studies, including Shaw *et al.*'s (1994a) study of toddlers from low-income families. Both Shaw *et al.* (1994a) and Richman *et al.* (1982) found that adversity factors that most closely reflected family relationships (discord and depression) were the strongest predictors of conduct problems, whereas chronic poverty showed inconsistent or no relationships with conduct problems (Pagani *et al.* 1999), suggesting that family dysfunction has a greater influence on child antisocial behaviour than material poverty. It is assumed that adversity factors act to make parenting more difficult, and that parenting is the common pathway through which these adversities impinge on young children's behaviour. There is evidence that good parenting, along with other factors such as the child's gender and temperament, may help to buffer the effects of adverse social circumstances on conduct problems (Rutter 1978; Sanson *et al.* 1991; Shaw *et al.* 1994a; Pettit *et al.* 1997).

Implications for intervention

From numerous studies which have employed the kinds of research design described above, we can draw the very broad conclusion that parenting has a powerful influence on child conduct problems, although it is by no means the only influence. It follows that interventions based on teaching parenting skills are likely to be successful, and indeed numerous randomised controlled trials show that this is the case, at least where interventions are based on behavioural and cognitive–behavioural principles. Moreover, some trials show that using these interventions alone, child problem behaviour can be reduced even in families who are experiencing other social problems such as depression (Webster-Stratton 1994), marital discord, and poverty (Sanders *et al.* in press). If good parenting helps to buffer the effects of social circumstances on conduct problems, then we would expect that parenting interventions would help ameliorate some social adversities. There is some evidence to support this notion, although this is likely to depend on the type and severity of problem. Webster-Stratton (1990) found that her parenting intervention improved maternal depression as well as child conduct problems, but had no beneficial effect on marital communication, suggesting it may be necessary and effective to intervene directly with these risk factors as well as teach parenting skills (Webster-Stratton 1994; Webster-Stratton and Hammond 1999).

The next sections examine studies that attempt to identify the key parenting mechanisms influencing child problem behaviour.

Patterson's coercion theory

Patterson (1982; Patterson *et al.* 1992) pioneered effective parenting interventions in tandem with basic observational research on family interaction. His coercion theory stresses that processes taking place during family conflict cause and maintain conduct problems. Antisocial behaviour is shaped and reinforced by thousands of episodes of conflict between family members. The difficult child learns to gain control over a chaotic or unpleasant family environment. He learns to avoid his parent's demands by persisting noisily with his own, whilst parent and sibs learn to give in. Both parent and child are negatively reinforced for their behaviour, by learning how to switch off the other's annoying behaviour. As the child learns the success of coercion, he may take this behaviour outside the home, where it may be reinforced by teachers or peers.

For a coercive interaction to start and perpetuate there may need to be a combination of a temperamentally difficult child and disrupted parenting skills, although Patterson's theory gives much greater weight to parenting mechanisms. His careful (1982) observational studies in the home found that compared to non-problem families, parents of children with conduct problems tended to be more harsh, erratic, and inconsistent in their responses to the child. Using robust measures from multiple settings and informants, Patterson *et al.* (1992) defined a set of 'family management' practices, including discipline, monitoring, and problem solving. Good discipline is defined as:

(i)   accurately tracking and noticing problem behaviour
(ii) ignoring trivial transgressions
(iii) having clear firm sanctions.

It is measured by direct observation, daily telephone interviews, and systematic observer ratings. Parent questionnaires did not correlate with other measures of discipline, so were not used in the main analyses. In three different longitudinal studies,

Patterson *et al.* (1992) found that poor discipline predicted the persistence of antisocial behaviour into adolescence, accounting for a highly significant 30% of the variance in antisocial outcomes, even after controlling for initial levels of antisocial behaviour. Patterson and Forgatch's (1995) intervention study found that the magnitude of improvement in parenting skill predicted the magnitude of improvement in 'harder' measures of antisocial behaviour at follow-up (e.g. arrest rates), providing evidence for a 'dose–response' relationship (Rutter 1994a) between discipline style and antisocial behaviour.

An important aspect of discipline that Patterson stresses, and which is a core skill in effective parent-training programmes, is for parents to follow through consistently on their demands to the child. However this behaviour is not directly measured and tested in his work. Gardner (1989) tested whether parents of conduct problem children were poorer at this. Systematic home observations showed that, compared to mothers in the control group, mothers of children with conduct problems were seven times more likely to be inconsistent by failing to follow through their demands during episodes of conflict. Moreover, the likelihood of the mother capitulating was significantly higher when the conflict began with a demand by the mother, compared to a demand by the child. This supports Patterson's negative reinforcement explanation that what children learn in conflictual families is to successfully avoid conforming with parental demands.

Implications Patterson's social learning theory model has stood up very well to the most rigorous causal tests yet seen in this field, especially for the parental discipline construct. The main implications for therapy are that this strongly affirms the importance of these basic discipline skills forming the core, though not necessarily the entirety, of any parenting intervention. These skills are very apparent in evidence-based interventions (e.g. Webster-Stratton *et al.* 1989, Webster-Stratton 1992; Tremblay *et al.* 1995; Sanders *et al.* in press) which teach parents to set consistent limits, follow through commands, ignore minor problems, and apply calm consequences such as time-out. Patterson's basic research and clinical trials suggest that parents of older children should also be taught monitoring and problem solving skills (Dishion *et al.* 1996). Despite evidence having been available for some years, few children receive this kind of therapy (Webster-Stratton and Taylor 1998), and many are offered different kinds of family and parenting interventions that have nothing like such a clear evidence base. It is important to point to the strength of the evidence in order to argue for more children getting this kind of help.

Limitations of coercion theory   Firstly, although parent-training has better evidence for its effectiveness than other therapies, the success rate could be higher. Patterson's data show that two-thirds of families are helped. There is evidence the success rate may be higher, up to 75%, in some pre-school samples (Webster-Stratton 1994). There is a need to improve this success rate, for example by drawing on other areas of basic research as well as social learning theory.

Secondly, Patterson's model argues that the most important thing to do is to help families to handle conflict and difficult behaviour better when it happens, in order to help the child to decrease his/her problem behaviour. However, many important parent–child interactions take place at other times, when there is no conflict. These encounters make up the great majority of interactions (Gardner 1987, 1994; Reid 1987), and it is likely that the nature of these more positive interactions influences when and whether conflict occurs, how it is resolved, and importantly, might give us clues as to how parents could help prevent problem behaviour from arising. These more positive interactions may be particularly important for the development of good relationships and the prevention of problem behaviour in younger children. Much of Patterson's model has been developed using older children, drawing little on basic developmental research. However, between early and middle childhood there are profound changes in relationships with parents and peers, and in moral development and social–cognitive skills, which may mean that different parenting mechanisms contribute to conduct problems at age 3 compared to age 10.

Studies of early positive interactions in the family

We will now look at some rather different theoretical approaches to understanding parent–child interaction, which focus less on clinical disorders and more on normal developmental processes, such as how parent and child build constructive, positive interactions. Recent studies have begun to examine how this basic research can help us understand the early development of conduct problems and their interventions (Pettit and Bates 1989; Zahn-Waxler *et al.* 1990; Gardner 1994; Shaw *et al.* 1994b; Campbell 1995; Pettit *et al.* 1997; Gardner *et al.* 1999a,b). Many of the same parenting constructs have been investigated in relation to conscience development, as will be discussed in a later section.

Playful interactions A number of studies have examined the influence of positive interactions such as joint play. Patterson *et al.* (1992) argue that these are not an important causal influence on behaviour problems, since their longitudinal studies found that parental positive behaviour accounted for little of the variance in conduct problems. But these studies measured only a limited range of variables, and this finding is at odds with many other studies. Patterson claims that where parents and conduct problem children have few harmonious interactions then this is a result, not a cause, of many years of problem behaviour.

However, Gardner (1987) found that observed rates of mother–child play and conversation were much lower in conduct problem than non-problem dyads, even at the ages of 3 and 4. Children with conduct problems instead spent more time in conflict, watching TV, and doing nothing. These findings suggest that children with conduct problems might be learning something different even when not engaged in conflict, as they were getting few models of cooperative, harmonious interaction with others. At this young age, low levels of positive interactions cannot easily be explained as resulting from years of conflict as Patterson (1982) suggests. Further support comes from a longitudinal study by Pettit and Bates (1989), who found that infrequent joint play in normal toddlers predicted 4-year-old problem behaviour.

These studies raise the question of what aspects of interaction during joint play are important. Accordingly, Gardner (1994) examined in detail the quality of interaction during joint play. She found that mothers of conduct problem children showed less warmth and more negative affect, were less responsive to their child's suggestions and questions, used less sensitive forms of control, and were less likely to initiate play. Once play had begun, mothers in the conduct problem group seemed to be less involved; they made fewer suggestions and asked fewer questions. In contrast, control group mothers made many more suggestions than their child and appeared to be in charge of the game, albeit in a more sensitive, warm, responsive manner. It might be argued that these patterns of maternal behaviour with conduct problem children were simply a reaction to trying to play with a negative, uncooperative child. But this seems an unlikely explanation, since the children were not especially difficult during play, and more group differences were found in mothers' behaviour than in children's. Thus children with conduct problems, compared to control group children, showed no higher rates of negative affect, and were actually more responsive to their mothers' suggestions than their mothers were to theirs. They made a good contribution to initiating and keeping the play going. These results are at least suggestive that positive parenting qualities during play may contribute to fewer conduct problems, rather than simply reflecting the child's effects on the parent in that situation. Other observational studies have come to similar conclusions. Pettit and Bates (1989) found that mothers who were involved and proactive during play had children with fewer behaviour problems. Shaw *et al.* (1994b) found that maternal responsiveness at age 1 predicted fewer behaviour problems at age 3 in boys only.

How do these findings match up with what is taught in parent training? Work with younger children by Forehand and McMahon (1981) and Webster-Stratton (1992; 1998) focuses on intervening first through joint play, and then teaching core discipline skills. They recommend regular play sessions, using praise, sensitive commands, warmth, and responding to the child's lead, just as basic research suggests. But they also place great emphasis on 'responsive play', where mothers exclusively follow the child's lead, not directing the play at all. In contrast, in Gardner's (1994) study, sitting back and letting the child take the lead was more characteristic of the mothers of problem children, whilst mothers in the control group took the lead a great deal. It is interesting that therapy teaches a style that does not entirely mirror that of normal parents. This raises the question of whether teaching 'responsive play' is the best strategy. Clinicians report that this technique appears effective at establishing warmer interactions. However, this element of the package of interventions has never been evaluated separately, so we don't know whether it is an essential component. It might be that the active ingredient is 'discipline' skill, or it might be that a different way of teaching play would work just as well. Alternatively, it could be that effective intervention strategies do not necessarily need to mimic normal good parenting. Where the relationship has become very negative, it may be helpful to teach unusually 'positive' strategies in order to rebuild the relationship.

Positive control strategies   What else does developmental research identify as predictors of good social adjustment in the pre-school years? Apart from playful interactions, the literature examines positive control strategies, (e.g. reasoning, negotiation, distraction, use of humour, and incentives) that are thought to help prevent and resolve conflict (Kuczynski 1984; Reid *et al.* 1994; Pettit *et al.* 1997; Gardner *et al.* 1999a,b). Some correlational, longitudinal, and experimental studies have been carried out, but few with clinical groups (Grusec and Goodnow 1994). These control strategies may operate through a number of possible mechanisms, such as by capturing the child's interest, giving him responsibility for his behaviour, showing the parent's interest in the child's viewpoint, and using a non-confrontational style (Dunn and Kendrick 1982; Grusec and Goodnow 1994). Kochanska and Aksan (1995) observed a cluster of maternal 'gentle' control strategies (e.g. reasoning, compromise, polite requests) that correlated positively with compliance in normal toddlers. Kuczynski's (1983, 1984) laboratory experiments show that reasoning can influence children's behaviour, but do not answer the question of whether parents' use of these strategies in natural settings can help prevent conduct problems.

We examined the contribution of positive strategies to conduct problems in a sample of 52 3-year-olds drawn from the New Forest epidemiological study (Gardner *et al.* 1999a), compared to the non-problem group. Mothers and 3-year-olds were observed during a clear-up task at home, and followed up at age 5. We found, contrary to predictions from the literature, that there were no differences in the frequency of these gentle control strategies; in fact, if anything, there was a slight trend for mothers to use more of these strategies in the problem group.

To interpret this finding, we looked more closely at the data and found that the frequency of positive strategies was highly correlated with child non-compliance. It might be expected that, after controlling statistically for the amount of non-compliance, mothers in the control group would then show a greater tendency to use these strategies. However, after doing this, using analysis of covariance, there were still no group differences in the frequency of positive strategies. Certainly it didn't seem that positive control strategies were something that mothers of difficult children were poor at, or needed to be taught how to do. This is of course exactly what Patterson (1982) would have predicted. He suggests that reasoning during conflict simply reinforces non-compliance, and therefore the problem group mothers would be expected to do more of this. These findings are based on a small sample studied in one context, but were replicated, for reasoning and bargaining, in a second study which sampled several situations in the home (Gardner *et al.* 1999b).

Timing of strategies   Do we know what is important about discipline strategies? Perhaps reasoning and bargaining can be helpful, but only if parents follow through on the consequences of their strategies, as is taught in parent-training (Webster-Stratton 1992). Alternatively, maybe reasoning and other positive strategies are only effective in certain contexts, for example, before conflict has started. The issue of how parents time their strategies seems to have been paid little attention in the literature. Particularly effective parenting might involve anticipating when a situation is likely to be difficult and taking steps to prevent conflict arising. Parent training manuals rarely make explicit mention of teaching skills for anticipating and preventing conflict, apart from the work of Sanders and Dadds (1982). Evidence to support the influence of preventive strategies comes from a study of normal children by Holden (1983), who examined parental anticipation using an elegant combination of observation in a supermarket, and experiment in the laboratory (Holden and West 1989). Both studies found that parents who took steps to prevent conflict by engaging the child before trouble occurred experienced less misbehaviour.

There appear to be good grounds for examining the timing of mothers' positive strategies and their relation to problems. In the study described earlier, Gardner *et al.* (1999a), it was hypothesised that:

(a) mothers of non-problem children would be more likely to offer a reason or incentive for clearing-up at the outset of the task, before the child started to misbehave. This was called a pre-emptive strategy.

(b) mothers of children with conduct problems would be more likely to wait till child had refused to tidy, then start to cajole them. This was called a reactive strategy.

The results showed that, although most mothers used reactive strategies, pre-emptive strategies were nevertheless used more often by mothers in the control group. A follow-up of half the sample found that mothers' use of pre-emptive strategies predicted fewer conduct problems at age 5, even after controlling for level of conduct problems at age 3. These longitudinal findings need interpreting with caution as the sample size was small. However, factors such as social class and maternal depression did not account for the links between pre-emptive strategies and conduct problems.

This study suggests that mothers of children with conduct problems have no difficulty using a range of positive discipline strategies to get their 3-year-old to clear up. However, group differences lay not in the content of strategies, but in their pre-emptive timing. Few studies have attempted to observe parents' preventive strategies, and this study suggests that it is possible to measure these by setting up everyday situations in the home which the parent knows in advance are going to happen, and which are likely to provoke mild conflict. If the finding of this study is replicated in a wider range of situations in the home, then this would be a good argument for putting the explicit teaching of pre-emptive strategies into intervention studies. It would be important to then test whether this component of the intervention actually makes a difference, as it would not be helpful to add components drawn from basic research without also testing their clinical value, using randomised controlled trials.

Parenting and conscience development

The literature on conscience or internalisation of values, like that on conduct problems, has examined the strategies parents use to promote positive behaviour and deal with conflict, as well as parents' overall style of interacting. The study of parenting and conscience is, however, less well developed than the study of parenting and conduct problems. Many studies have used interview rather than observational methods. Where longitudinal designs are used, they rarely take account of the child's initial level of conscience development when examining how parenting style at one time point contributes to later child outcomes. Finally, since much of this literature comes from the study of normal development rather than clinical problems, there is no body of experimental intervention literature to help test the causal influence of parenting on conscience.

Developmental psychologists have been studying the influences on children's moral development for many years. However, the influence of Piaget (1932) and Kohlberg (1969), who argued that children develop an understanding of morality through a series of stages, led to a neglect of the influences of parenting in the early years. However, in recent years there has been a resurgence of interest in emotional aspects of morality (e.g. Eisenberg and Miller 1987) and on moral behaviour rather than reasoning (e.g. Kochanska 1993). It has therefore been recognised that even young children demonstrate an awareness of moral issues, and hence researchers have begun to study the origins of conscience in early childhood.

Much developmental research has focused on the factors which influence a child to take on the values of their parents and society as if they were their own, which is often termed 'internalisation'. One of the earliest studies of the influences of parenting on internalisation was conducted by Sears *et al.* (1957). Interviewing a large sample of mothers, they distinguished between two forms of discipline. The first, termed 'love-oriented', included praise, social isolation, love withdrawal, and reasoning. The second form, 'object-oriented', included tangible rewards, deprivation of goods and privileges, and physical punishment. They found that love withdrawal by warm mothers was a particularly effective method of promoting internalisation. Hoffman (1970, 1983) studied parental reports of their behaviour in discipline and control situations. He distinguished between power assertive strategies (physical punishment, deprivation of objects or privileges, use of force or threats), love withdrawal (direct but non-physical expression of disapproval or anger), and use of reasoning (explanations, appeals to children's pride). He found that there was a tendency for internalisation to be negatively related to power assertion and positively related to reasoning. Hoffman (1983) argued that excessive power assertion

(a) provokes anger in the child;
(b) provides a model for the antisocial discharge of anger;
(c) focuses the child's attention on the self rather than the object of harm;
(d) increases arousal and reduces a child's ability to process information about the situation;
(e) fails to take advantage of the child's natural empathic abilities.

Nevertheless, Hoffman (1983) also argued that a certain minimal amount of power assertion may help capture the child's attention so that the reason can be efficiently processed. This work echoes that of Baumrind (1967, 1971), who argued that the optimum parenting style was one which included both high levels of warmth and high levels of control. Thus both Baumrind and Hoffman suggest that a certain amount of power assertion is necessary for motivation. It should be noted that these theories were developed with reference to late childhood and early adolescence, when the foundations for moral development have already been established. Data on parenting behaviours was also gathered by interview rather than direct observation. However, part of Hoffman's hypothesis is supported by an observational study which found that pre-schoolers whose mothers used reasoning and humanistic conflict resolution had higher levels of moral understanding at ages 6 and 7 (Dunn *et al.* 1995).

More recent work has focused on the origins of conscience in early childhood. In particular, Kochanska (1993, 1997a,b) has developed robust multiple measures of conscience. These include a maternal questionnaire (Kochanska *et al.* 1994), a child narrative task to assess understanding of moral issues (Kochanska *et al.* 1996), and ingenious techniques for observing child with parent, alone with forbidden toys, and participating in tasks such as cheating games (Kochanska *et al.* 1995). Parenting is observed directly in interactions with the child in structured situations and longitudinal designs are used to determine what parenting factors influence the development of conscience over time (e.g. Kochanska *et al.* 1995; Kochanska 1997a,b). Kochanska's research on young children has confirmed some of the findings of researchers such as Hoffman, in that conscience appears to be negatively related to use of power assertion (Kochanska 1991; Kochanska *et al.* 1996). On the other hand, shared positive affect (warmth) appears to be particularly important for the development of conscience, perhaps because of motivational factors (Kochanska and Aksan 1995; Kochanska *et al.* 1995; Kochanska 1997b). This work suggests interesting avenues for research into the development of conscience in young children with conduct problems. Only one study has examined early signs of conscience development (e.g. empathy, helping) in children at risk for behaviour problems (Zahn-Waxler *et al.* 1994). Their findings did not show a clear inverse relationship between conduct problems and conscience development, and gender differences were also observed. More longitudinal studies are needed to establish how the relationship between conscience and conduct problems develops over time. In particular, further research should examine the adolescent and adult outcomes of different levels of conscience development, in terms of moral development, covert and overt conduct problems, and later antisocial personality.

To a certain extent, this work is consistent with much of the literature on parenting and the development of conduct problems. Both the developmental and clinical literature indicate that whilst a certain amount of firm and consistent discipline is necessary, excessive amounts of power assertion and angry behaviour have negative consequences. With regard to non-conflict situations, both literatures indicate that a warm and nurturing relationship with a parent encourages the child to adopt parental values. Furthermore, parental expression of disapproval, in a non-threatening manner during conflict, appears to be more effective if it occurs within the context of a warm and supportive, rather than combative, relationship. However, the role of reasoning is less consistent between the two literatures. Social learning theory (Bandura 1977; Patterson 1982) would predict that reasoning used during conflict reinforces a child's misbehaviour as they are receiving parental attention. The implication that parental rules and standards are negotiable could be seen as negative in the sense of indicating parents have unclear boundaries, but a more positive interpretation is that reasoning reflects parental willingness to understand the child's perspective. Research described earlier on timing of strategies (Gardner *et al.* 1999a,b) offers an alternative explanation, namely that reasoning may only be effective in certain contexts, for example, when used before any potential conflict has arisen. This maximises the likelihood that the child will pay attention to the message, because he is not over-aroused and neither is he positively reinforced for misbehaviour. It is possible that clinicians have been unwilling to include use of reasoning in parent training programmes, because if used excessively it could detract from parents' use of clear and simple commands. However, developmental literature provides good evidence that use of reasoning promotes children's long-term socialisation and conscience development, which may help prevent serious outcomes of conduct disorder in adolescence. It is essential that children learn to take responsibility for their own behaviour, and evidence suggests that this process begins at a very young age. In terms of parenting interventions, it may be more appropriate to encourage parents to promote this sense of autonomy in their child at a later stage of intervention, after standards for acceptable behaviour have been established. In summary therefore, there is a high level of consistency between literature on moral development and research on conduct disorder, particularly with reference to power assertion and warmth of the parent–child relationship. However, parent training programmes presently neglect the importance of parenting strategies which encourage a child to take responsibility for their own behaviour. Recognition of this work may lead to improved long-term outcomes for children with conduct problems.

Conclusions

First, the research on conduct problems reviewed in this chapter shows clearly the importance of Patterson's parental discipline skills in the development and treatment of children's antisocial behaviour. The evidence from a substantial body of longitudinal studies and controlled therapy trials suggests that these skills need to form the core of any parenting intervention. There are, however, other more positive parenting skills, including play skills and positive control strategies, which recent evidence suggests may be critical, particularly in the early development of conduct problems, and which form a component of some parenting interventions. Basic research has begun to identify some strategies that parents use to prevent problem behaviour. These strategies may be particularly important, and warrant further testing in longitudinal studies, followed by careful testing in the context of well-controlled intervention trials. This may serve the twin purposes of helping to improve the outcome of therapy, and further testing theories about the precise parenting mechanisms which contribute to the development of these very common and serious disorders in children.

Second, although research on the effects of parenting on conscience is less well developed than that on conduct problems, it appears to be a promising area for investigation. Notably, it is based on a body of developmental theory which examines not only behavioural manifestations of conscience, but also attempts to measure directly, and to make inferences about, the child's internal cognitive state, using concepts such as empathy, moral awareness, and internalisation. A well-developed conscience can be seen as something the child carries with him, and that promotes resilience in the face of adverse circumstances, for example peer pressure to vandalise or steal. The studies reviewed suggest there are parenting strategies and styles that influence conscience development in young children, and many of these also appear to influence the development of conduct problems. Before we can tell if these could be translated into prevention approaches, a number of steps are needed. Firstly, we need to know whether poor early conscience development contributes to the prediction of later conduct problems, and to the prediction of severe or psychopathic antisocial behaviour. Longitudinal studies are needed which examine conscience development at different stages in a sample of children at high risk for conduct disorder. Secondly we need to test further the causal contribution of parenting to conscience using longitudinal and experimental studies. The third stage would depend on these findings, and would require very large-scale studies as some of the outcomes are rare, and take many years to develop. It would involve developing early preventive approaches and carrying out rigorous trials to examine their effects on conduct problems and on antisocial personality disorder.

References

American Psychiatric Association (1994). *Diagnostic and statistical manual of mental disorders*. 4th edn. Washington, DC, American Psychiatric Association.

Bandura, A. (1977). *Social learning theory*. Englewood Cliffs, NJ, Prentice Hall.

Barlow, J. (1998). Parent-training programmes and behaviour problems—findings from a systematic review. In A. Buchanan and B. L. Hudson (eds.), *Parenting, schooling and children's behaviour*. Aldershot, Ashgate, pp. 89–110.

Bates, J. E., Bayles, K., Bennett, D. S., *et al.* (1991). Origins of externalizing behavior problems at eight years of age. In D. J. Pepler and K. Rubin (eds.), *The development and treatment of childhood aggression*, pp. 93–120. Hillsdale, NJ, Erlbaum.

Baumrind, D. (1967). Child care practices anteceding three patterns of pre-school behavior. *Genetic Psychology Monographs*, **75**, 43–88.

Baumrind, D. (1971). Current patterns of parental authority. *Developmental Psychology Monographs*, **4**, 1–101.

120   *Promoting children's emotional well-being*

Bryant, P. E. (1985). Parents, children and cognitive development. In R. A. Hinde, A. Clermont, and J. Stevenson-Hinde (eds.), *Social Relationships and Cognitive Development*, pp. 239–52.

Campbell, S. B. (1995). Behavior problems in pre-school children: a review of recent research. *Journal of Child Psychology and Psychiatry*, **36**, 113–49.

Capaldi, D. M. and Clark, S. (1998). Prospective family predictors of aggression toward female partners for at-risk young men. *Developmental Psychology*, **34**, 1175–88.

Capaldi, D. M. and Stoolmiller, M. (1999). Co-occurrence of conduct problems and depressive symptoms in early adolescent boys: III. Prediction to young-adult adjustment. *Development and Psychopathology*, **11**, 59–84.

Cunningham, C., Bremner, R., and Boyle, M. (1995). Large group community-based parenting programs for families of preschoolers at risk for disruptive behaviour disorders: utilization, cost effectiveness and outcome. *Journal of Child Psychology and Psychiatry*, **36**, 1141–60.

Deater-Deckard, K., Dodge, K. A., Bates, J. E., and Pettit, G. S. (1996). Physical discipline among African American and European American mothers: links to children's externalizing behaviors. *Developmental Psychology*, **32**, 1065–72.

Deater-Deckard, K. and Plomin, R. (in press). An adoption study of the etiology of teacher and parent reports of externalizing behavior problems in middle childhood. *Child Development*.

Dishion, T. J., Patterson, G. R., and Kavanagh, K. A. (1992). An experimental test of the coercion model: linking theory, measurement, and intervention. In J. McCord and R. E. Tremblay (eds), *Preventing antisocial behavior: interventions from birth through adolescence*, pp. 253–82. New York, Guilford.

Dishion, T. J., French, D. C., and Patterson, G. R. (1995). The development and ecology of antisocial behavior. In D. Cicchetti and D. Cohen (eds.), *Developmental psychopathology*, pp. 421–70. Vol. **2**. New York, Wiley.

Dishion, T. J., Andrews, D. W., Kavanagh, K., and Soberman, L. (1996). Preventive interventions for high-risk youth: the Adolescent Transitions Program. In R. Peters and R. J. McMahon (eds.), *Preventing childhood disorders, substance abuse, and delinquency*, pp. 184–214. Thousand Oaks, CA, Sage.

Dumas, J. E., LaFreniere, P. J., and Serketich, W. J. (1995). 'Balance of power': a transactional analysis of control in mother-child dyads involving socially competent aggressive, and anxious children. *Journal of Abnormal Psychology*, **104**, 104–13.

Dunn, J. and Kendrick, C. (1982). *Siblings: love, envy and understanding*. London, Grant McIntyre.

Dunn, J., Brown, J. R., and Maguire, M. (1995). The development of children's moral sensibility: individual differences and emotion understanding. *Developmental Psychology*, **31**, 649–59.

Eaves, L. J., Silberg, J. L., Meyer, J. M., *et al.* (1997). Genetics and developmental psychopathology: 2. The main effects of genes and environment on behavioral problems in the Virginia Twin Study of adolescent behavioral development. *Journal of Child Psychology and Psychiatry*, **38**, 965–80.

Eisenberg, N. and Miller, P. A. (1987). The relation of empathy to prosocial and related behaviours. *Psychological Bulletin*, **101**, 91–119.

Fergusson, D. M. and Horwood, L. J. (1998). Early conduct problems and later life opportunities. *Journal of Child Psychology and Psychiatry*, **39**, 1097–108.

Fergusson, D. M. and Lynskey, M. T. (1998). Conduct problems in childhood and psychosocial outcomes in young adulthood: a prospective study. *Journal of Emotional and Behavioral Disorders*, **6**, 2–18.

Forehand, R. L. and McMahon, R. J. (1981). *Helping the noncompliant child*. NY, Guilford.

Forgatch, M. S. (1991). The clinical science vortex: a developing theory of antisocial behavior. In D. J. Pepler and K. H. Rubin (eds.), *Development and treatment of childhood aggression*, pp. 291–315. Hillsdale, NJ, Erlbaum.

Frick, P. J., Lahey, B. B., Loeber, R., *et al.* (1993). Oppositional defiant disorder and conduct disorder: a meta-analytic view of factor analyses and cross-validation in a clinic sample. *Clinical Psychology Review*, **13**, 319–40.

Frick, P. J., O'Brien, B. S., Wootton, J. M., and McBurnett, K. (1994). Psychopathy and conduct problems in children. *Journal of Abnormal Psychology*, **103**, 700–7.

Gardner, F. (1987). Positive interaction between mothers and children with conduct problems: is there training for harmony as well as fighting? *Journal of Abnormal Child Psychology*, **15**, 283–93.

Gardner, F. (1989). Inconsistent parenting: is there evidence for a link with children's conduct problems? *Journal of Abnormal Child Psychology*, **17**, 223–33.

Gardner, F. (1994). The quality of joint activity between mothers and their children with behaviour problems. *Journal of Child Psychology and Psychiatry*, **35**, 935–48.

Gardner, F. (1997). Observational methods for recording parent–child interaction: how generalisable are the findings? *Child Psychology and Psychiatry Review*, **2**(2), 70–75.

Gardner, F., Sonuga-Barke, E., and Sayal, K. (1999a). Parents anticipating misbehavior: an observational study of strategies parents use to prevent conflict with behavior problem children. *Journal of Child Psychology and Psychiatry*, **40**, 1185–96.

Gardner, F., Burton, J., and Wilson, C. (1999b). *Positive parenting style:*

how does it influence the early development of conduct problems? Paper presented at International Society for Research in Child and Adolescent Psychopathology, Barcelona, June 1999.

Gjone, H. and Stevenson, J. (1997). The association between internalizing and externalizing behavior in childhood and early adolescence: genetic or common environmental influences? *Journal of Abnormal Child Psychology*, **25**, 277–86.

Grusec, J. E. and Goodnow, J. J. (1994). Impact of parental discipline methods on the child's internalization of values: a reconceptualization of current points of view. *Developmental Psychology*, **30**, 4–19.

Hare, R. D., Hart, S. D., and Harpur, T. J. (1991). Psychopathy and the DSM criteria for antisocial personality disorder. *Journal of Abnormal Psychology*, **100**, 391–8.

Harpur, T. J., Hare, R. D., and Hakistan, A. R. (1989). Two factor conceptualisation of psychopathy: construct validity and assessment implications. *Psychological Assessment*, **1**, 6–17.

Health Advisory Service (1995). *Together we Stand*. London, HMSO.

Hoffman, M. L. (1970). Moral development. In P. H. Mussen (ed.), *Carmichael's manual of child psychology*, pp. 261–360. NY, Wiley.

Hoffman, M. L. (1975). Moral internalisation, parental power, and the nature of parent–child interaction. *Developmental Psychology*, **11**, 228–39.

Hoffman, M. L. (1983). Affective and cognitive processes in moral internalisation. In E. T. Higgins, D. Ruble, and W. Hartup (eds.), *Social cognition and social development: a socio-cultural perspective*, pp. 236–24. Cambridge, Cambridge University Press.

Holden, G. W. (1983). Avoiding conflict: mothers as tacticians in the supermarket. *Child Development*, **54**, 233–40.

Holden, G. W. and West, M. J. (1989). Proximate regulation by mothers: a demonstration of how differing styles affect young children's behavior. *Child Development*, **60**, 64–9.

Kazdin, A. E. (1993). Treatment of conduct disorder: progress and directions in psychotherapy research. *Development and Psychopathology*, **5**, 277–310.

Kochanska, G. (1991). Socialisation and temperament in the development of guilt and conscience. *Child Development*, **62**, 1379–92.

Kochanska, G. (1993). Toward a synthesis of parental socialisation and child temperament in early development of conscience. *Child Development*, **64**, 325–47.

Kochanska, G. (1997a). Mutually positive orientation between mothers and their young children: implications for early socialisation. *Child Development*, **68**, 94–112.

Kochanska, G. (1997b). Multiple pathways to conscience for children with different temperaments: from toddlerhood to age 5. *Developmental Psychology*, **33**, 228–40.

Kochanska, G. and Aksan, N. (1995). Mother-child mutually positive affect, the quality of child compliance to requests and prohibitions, and maternal control as correlates of early internalization. *Child Development*, **66**, 236–54.

Kochanska, G., Kuczynski, L., and Radke-Yarrow, M. (1989). Correspondence between mother's self-reported and observed child rearing practices. *Child Development*, **60**, 56–63.

Kochanska, G., DeVet, K., Goldman, M., *et al.* (1994). Maternal reports of conscience development and temperament in young children. *Child Development*, **65**, 852–68.

Kochanska, G., Aksan, N., and Koenig, A. L. (1995). A longitudinal study of the roots of preschooler's conscience: committed compliance and emerging internalisation. *Child Development*, **66**, 1752–70.

Kochanska, G., Padavich, D. L., and Koenig, A. (1996). Children's narratives about hypothetical moral dilemmas and objective measures of their conscience: mutual relations and socialization antecedents. *Child Development*, **67**, 1420–36.

Kohlberg, L. (1969). Stage and sequence: the cognitive-developmental approach to socialization. In D. Goslin (ed.), *The handbook of socialization theory and research*, pp. 347–479. Chicago, Rand McNally.

Kuczynski, L. (1983). Reasoning, prohibitions, and motivations for compliance. *Developmental Psychology*, **19**, 126–34.

Kuczynski, L. (1984). Socialization goals and mother-child interaction: strategies for long-term and short-term compliance. *Developmental Psychology*, **20**, 1061–73.

Loeber, R. (1990). Development and risk factors of juvenile antisocial behavior and delinquency. *Clinical Psychology Review*, **10**, 1–41.

Loeber, R., and Farrington, D. P. (1994). Problems and solutions in longitudinal and experimental treatment studies of child psychopathology and delinquency. *Journal of Consulting and Clinical Psychology*, **62**, 887–900.

Loeber, R., and Hay, D. (1994). Developmental approaches to aggression and conduct problems. In M. L. Rutter and D. Hay (eds.), *Development through life: a handbook for clinicians*, pp. 488–516. Oxford, Blackwell.

Loeber, R., Wung, P., Keenan, K., *et al.* (1993). Developmental pathways in disruptive child behaviour. *Development and Psychopathology*, **5**, 103–33.

Loeber, R., Keenan, K., and Zhang, Q. (1997). Boys' experimentation and persistence in developmental pathways toward serious delinquency. *Journal of Abnormal Child Psychology*, **13**, 337–52.

Maccoby, E. E. and Martin, J. A. (1983). Socialization in the context of the family: parent–child interaction. In E. M. Hetherington (ed.), *Handbook of child psychology: Vol. 4, Socialization, personality and social development*, pp. 1–101. New York, Wiley.

Miller, P. A., and Eisenberg, N. (1988). The relation of empathy to aggression and externalising/antisocial behaviour. *Psychological Bulletin*, **103**, 324–44.

Moffitt, T. E. and Caspi, A. (1998). Implications of violence between intimate partners for child psychologists and psychiatrists. *Journal of Child Psychology and Psychiatry*, **39**, 137–44.

Pagani, L., Boulerice, B., Vitaro, F., and Tremblay, R. E. (1999). Effects of poverty on academic failure and delinquency in boys: a change and process model approach. *Journal of Child Psychology and Psychiatry*, **40**, 1209–19.

Patrick, C. J., Zempolich, K. A., and Levenston, G. K. (1997). Emotionality and violent behaviour in psychopaths: a biosocial analysis. In A. Raine, P. Brennan, D. P. Farrington, and S. A. Mednick (eds.), *Biosocial bases of violence*, pp. 145–63. New York, Plenum.

Patterson, G. R. (1982). *Coercive family process*. Eugene, OR, Castalia. (Chapter 3: Observations of family process.)

Patterson. G. R. and Forgatch, M. S. (1995). Predicting future clinical adjustment from treatment outcome and process variables. *Psychological Assessment*, **7**, 275–85.

Patterson, G. R., Reid, J. B., and Dishion, T. J. (1992). *Antisocial boys*. Eugene, OR, Castalia.

Pettit, G. S. and Bates, J. E. (1989). Family interaction patterns and children's behavior problems from infancy to four years. *Developmental Psychology*, **25**, 413–20.

Pettit, G. S., Bates, J. E., and Dodge, K. E. (1997). Supportive parenting, ecological context, and children's adjustment: a seven-year longitudinal study. *Child Development*, **68**, 908–23.

Piaget, J. (1932/1965). *The moral judgement of the child*. New York, Academic.

Plomin, R. (1994). The Emmanuel Miller Memorial Lecture 1993. Genetic research and identification of environmental influences. *Journal of Child Psychology and Psychiatry*, **35**, 817–34.

Plomin, R., Nitz, K., and Rowe, D. (1990). Behavioral genetics and aggressive behavior in childhood. In M. Lewis and S. M. Miller (eds.), *Handbook of developmental psychopathology: perspectives in developmental psychology*, pp. 119–33. New York, Plenum.

Reid, J. B. (1978). *A social learning approach to family intervention. Vol II: Observation in home settings*. Eugene, OR: Castalia.

Reid, J. B. (1987). Social interactional patterns in families of abused and nonabused children. In C. Zahn-Waxler, M. Cummings, and R. Ianotti (eds.), *Altruism and aggression: biological and social origins*. Cambridge, Cambridge University Press.

Reid, J. B. (1993). Prevention of conduct disorder before and after school entry: relating interventions to developmental findings, *Journal of Development and Psychopathology*. **5**, 243–62.

Reid, M. J., O'Leary, S. G., and Wolff, L. S. (1994). Effects of maternal distraction and reprimands on toddlers' transgressions and negative affect. *Journal of Abnormal Child Psychology*, **22**, 237–46.

Richman, N., Stevenson, J., and Graham, P. (1982). *Pre-school to school: a behavioural study*. London, Academic.

Robins, L. N. (1991). Conduct disorder. *Journal of Child Psychology and Psychiatry*, **32**, 193–212.

Robins, L. N., Tipp, J., and McEvoy, L. (1991). Antisocial personality. In L. N. Robins and D. Regier (eds.), *Psychiatric disorders in America*. New York, Free Press.

Rutter, M. (1978). Family, area and school influences in the genesis of conduct disorders. In L. A. Hersov, D. Berger, and D. Shaffer (eds.), *Aggression and anti-social behaviour in childhood and adolescence*, pp. 95–113. Oxford, Pergamon.

Rutter, M. (1994a). Beyond longitudinal data: causes, consequences, changes, and continuity. *Journal of Consulting and Clinical Psychology*, **62**, 928–40.

Rutter, M. (1994b). Family discord and conduct disorder: cause, consequence, or correlate? *Journal of Family Psychology*, **8**, 170–86.

Rutter, M., Silberg, J., O'Connor, T., and Simonoff, E. (1999). Genetics and child psychiatry: II Empirical research findings. *Journal of Child Psychology and Psychiatry*, **40**, 19–55.

Rydelius, P. A. (1988). The development of antisocial behaviour and sudden violent death. *Acta Psychiatrica Scandanavica*, **77**, 398–403.

Sanders, M. R. and Dadds, M. R. (1982). Effects of planned activities and child management procedures in parent training: an analysis of setting generality. *Behavior Therapy*, **13**, 452–61.

Sanders, M. R., Markie-Dadds, C., Tully, L. A., and Bor, W. (in press). The Triple P-Positive Parenting Program: a comparison of enhanced, standard and self-directed behavioral family intervention for parents of children with early onset conduct problems. *Journal of Consulting and Clinical Psychology*.

Sanson, A., Oberklaid, F., Pedlow, R., and Prior, M. (1991). Risk indicators: assessment of infancy predictors of pre-school behavioural maladjustment. *Journal of Child Psychology and Psychiatry*, **32**, 609–26.

Schaffer, H. R. (1996). *Social development*. Oxford, Blackwell. (Chapter 6: From Other-control to Self-control.)

Schwartz, D, McFadyen-Ketchum, S., Dodge, K., and Pettit, G. (1999). Early behavior problems as predictor of later peer group victimization: moderators and mediators in the pathways of social risk. *Journal of Abnormal Child Psychology*, **27**, 191–203.

Sears, R. R., Maccoby, E. E., and Levin, H. (1957). *Patterns of child rearing*. New York, Harper and Row.

Serketich, W. J., and Dumas, J. E. (1996). The effectiveness of behavioral parent training to modify antisocial behavior in children: a meta-analysis. *Behavior Therapy*, **27**, 171–86.

Shaw, D. S., Vondra, J. I., Hommerding, K. D., *et al.* (1994a). Chronic family adversity and early child behavior problems: a longitudinal study of low income families. *Journal of Child Psychology and Psychiatry*, **35**, 1109–22.

Shaw, D. S., Keenan, K., and Vondra, J. I. (1994b). Developmental precursors of externalizing behavior: ages 1 to 3. *Developmental Psychology*, **30**, 355–64.

Shaw, D. S., Winslow, E. B., Owens, E. B., *et al.* (1998). The development of early externalizing problems among children from low-income families: a transformational perspective. *Journal of Abnormal Child Psychology*, **26**, 95–107.

Simonoff, E., Pickles, A., Hewitt, J., *et al.* (1995). Multiple raters of disruptive child behavior; using a genetic strategy to examine shared views and bias. *Behavior Genetics*, **25**, 311–26.

Taylor, T. K. and Biglan, A. (1998). Behavioral family interventions for improving child- rearing: a review of the literature for practitioners and policy makers. *Clinical Child and Family Psychology Review*, **1**, 41–60.

Tremblay, R. E., Pagani-Kurtz, L., Masse, L. C., *et al.* (1995). A bimodal preventive intervention for disruptive kindergarten boys: its impact through mid-adolescence. *Journal of Consulting and Clinical Psychology*, **63**, 560–8.

Webster-Stratton, C. (1990). Long term follow up of families with young conduct problem children: from pre-school to grade school. *Journal of Clinical Child Psychology* **19**, 144–9.

Webster-Stratton, C. (1992). *The incredible years: a trouble-shooting guide for parents of children ages 3–8 years*. Toronto, Umbrella.

Webster-Stratton, C. (1994). Advancing videotape parent training: a comparison study. *Journal of Consulting and Clinical Psychology*, **62**, 583–93.

Webster-Stratton, C. (1998). Preventing conduct problems in head start children: strengthening parenting competences. *Journal of Consulting and Clinical Psychology*, **66**, 715–30.

Webster-Stratton, C. and Hammond, M. (1999). Marital conflict management skills, parenting style, and early-onset conduct problems: processes and pathways. *Journal of Child Psychology and Psychiatry*, **40**, 917–27.

Webster-Stratton, C. and Spitzer, A. (1991). Development, reliability, and validity of the daily telephone discipline interview. *Behavioral Assessment*, **13**, 221–39.

Webster-Stratton, C. and Taylor, T. K. (1998). Adopting and implementing empirically supported interventions: a recipe for success. In A. Buchanan and B. L. Hudson (eds.), *Parenting, schooling and children's behaviour*. Aldershot, Ashgate, pp. 127–161.

Webster-Stratton, C., Kolpacoff, M., and Hollinsworth, T. (1989). The long-term effectiveness and clinical significance of three cost-effective training programs for families with conduct problem children. *Journal of Consulting and Clinical Psychology*, **57**, 550–3.

White, J. L., Moffitt, T. E., Earls, F., *et al.* (1990). How early can we tell? Predictors of childhood conduct disorder and adolescent delinquency. *Criminology*, **28**, 507–28.

Zahn-Waxler, C., Iannotti, R. J., Cummings, E. M., and Denham, S. (1990). Antecedents of problem behaviors in children of depressed mothers. *Development and Psychopathology*, **2**, 271–91.

Zahn-Waxler, C., Cole, P. M., Richardson, D. T., *et al.* (1994). Social problem solving in disruptive preschool children: reactions to hypothetical situations of conflict and distress. *Merrill-Palmer Quarterly*, **40**, 98–119.

6

Parenting programmes: the importance of partnership in research and practice

Roger Grimshaw

'Anything that anybody can give you that's reasonable you should listen to it even if you decide not to take on board the advice, so I mean, then you have the choice. Once you have the choice then it's down to you, not anybody else, and I am very much in favour of, you have to make your own decisions, no matter how many people you ask about something, at the end of the day, it's your choice as to what you do.' Parenting programme attender

Introduction

Ordinarily we think of human action as the fruit of decision. Social scientists are in the business of trying to understand decision making as something more than simply random and yet less than perfectly rational. They look to social processes to see how the substance and the scope of decision making are defined. They identify the ways in which an individual's goals of action are shaped by interaction with a whole range of social others. They wish to investigate the reference groups that hold effective sway over individual conduct and they study the means by which a particular group seeks to extend its influence over another's decisions.

In these respects decisions about parenting are no different from other decisions: they take place in a social context containing reference groups; attempts to understand, and attempts to influence decisions, are manifold, whether through commercial advertising, through professional assessment and advice, or through family conversations. Parenting programmes represent one of the most specific and determined endeavours of this kind that we have seen. Indeed pressures to demonstrate their impact have mounted as government agencies anxious about apparent family trends have sought to find mechanisms that can be shown to 'work' benignly. Getting 'results' implies a focus on selecting the 'right' programme message that duly learned and understood will lead to the desired outcomes. Yet too little attention has been paid to the social preconditions that influence participation in programmes and receptiveness to their messages.

In the USA the use of parenting programmes in public projects has been accompanied by an impressive commitment to evaluation aimed at determining their effects. In the UK parenting programmes have become a focus of attention from policy makers precisely because of this appealing determination to make an impact, and the evidence of key studies has encouraged a growing belief in their efficacy (Lloyd 1999). Nonetheless I will argue that where this influence on parents occurs it is not simple or unmediated. It depends on the capacity of programmes to work with parents in a spirit of *partnership* that confirms the parent as a decision maker.

In this chapter I want to clarify how parenting programmes relate to the goals of parents themselves and, in particular, to show how other parents form a key reference group for the individual. Only by taking into account this social dimension can programme organisers ensure that parents become not passive targets but active partners and stakeholders in the programmes. Such an approach should be reflected both in evaluative research and in the practice of helping parents.

First of all, I shall review key findings from the USA–UK literature in order to substantiate the points made so far. Then, to illustrate and expand the argument, I will draw on the evidence of a recent UK study that compared the perspectives and goals of major stakeholders in the programmes. Within the space available here it is not possible to do justice to other features of the UK study, particularly those relating to the development of children's conceptions of parenthood.

Searching for 'what works'

The attempt to arrive at a specification of effective programmes has been a feature of USA social policy and practice for some years, while in the UK interest in this approach has been growing more recently (Macdonald and Roberts 1995). Though programmes for parents vary in conceptualisation and approach, the disciplines of 'what works' have been most conspicuously applied to versions of 'parent training' using behavioural techniques that have attracted interest from clinicians looking for replicable and effective methods to deal with significant problems. However, we know more about the aggregate effectiveness of such methods than about whom they work best for. Nor do we understand fully the ways in which parents' goals and reference groups influence how these and other programmes work.

Goals, partnership, and outcomes

The importance of goals in parenting services has been well expressed by a recent author who argues that we should unpack issues of effectiveness into questions like 'What do the users/staff/funders think they *should be* doing?' (Smith 1998, p. 113 – emphasis in original.)

Indeed, collaboration with parents is a basic tenet of therapeutic work (Webster-Stratton and Herbert 1994). Parent training coordinators consult with parents about their goals before embarking on the training. Nonetheless, how far the approach used in these encounters lays the groundwork for a reliable and effective partnership will depend on several preconditions that seem to be related to social factors.

Although the literature attests to the effectiveness of parenting programmes in improving the behaviour of pre-adolescent children, the picture is not completely reassuring. A large proportion of parent attenders on successful programmes are unable to derive long-term benefits from them. Continued problems are more likely among parents who are single, from lower social strata, suffer from maternal depression, or have a family history of alcoholism and drug abuse (Webster-Stratton and Hammond 1990).

Broad reviews of the field have shown that recruitment tends to be from middle class parents and concentrated among mothers (Dembo *et al.* 1985; Medway 1989). In particular, recent reviews of parent training have shown significant rates of drop-out – at least a quarter of parents (Barlow 1998). Increasingly it is perceived that part of the answer to drop-out is to acknowledge the individual goals of parents from different cultural backgrounds (Webster-Stratton and Taylor 1998). It is essential to understand the complex modern process of 'enculturation' as families exposed to different cultures select options that suit their needs (Halstead 1994; Dosanjh and Ghuman 1998). Initiatives in the multi-cultural London borough of Newham have shown that, when programmes have been delivered in five languages other than English, participation can reach impressive levels (Samra 1999).

Parents want support

It seems that support is a critical element in any specification of parents' needs. Support groups are significantly welcomed by parents in need. A study of family centres in the UK showed that disadvantaged parents overwhelmingly wanted 'other adults to talk to' (Smith 1998, p. 118), while access to expert advice was a somewhat lower priority. A study of mothers with low birth weight babies showed that mothers valued groups almost as highly as family support (Oakley 1993). It is not surprising that groups have been chosen as attractive vehicles for the transmission of ideas about parenting.

Acknowledging the value of support means taking seriously the networks within a specific community. For example, the high value placed by parents on support from their peers has been recognised by attempts to train 'community mothers' who offer help to others in the same community (Johnson and Molloy 1995). The importance of creating services that are sensitive to the needs and outlooks of minority groups is reflected in a recent review of USA developments that cites evidence of some success in devising programmes used by inner city African–Americans (Long 1997). The same author has pointed to the need for consumer information that promotes awareness and choice.

Groups – the upside and the downside

Groups are potent mechanisms for delivering messages to parents and for helping them to reduce behavioural problems. A systematic review of evidence has shown that group pro-grammes can be more effective than individual programmes (Barlow 1997).

What is it that makes group programmes apparently more effective than individual services? It cannot be the message that makes a difference. It is more likely to be the power of the group to support the individual, to mirror concerns, and encourage achievement. Such effects may impact on the long-term future of families by reinforcing networks of help within localities and communities. Once again the social reference points of parents are implicated in the search for what really works.

Of course, groups are not passive instruments that can be manipulated at will. To accept the messages brought by pro-gramme coordinators, groups demand a form of address that is respectful and capable of speaking to the preoccupations of members. The use of the somewhat obscure term 'facilitator' to describe those who deliver programmes nonetheless reflects such demands in a way that is less visible in the literature that speaks of 'therapy', 'education', or 'training'. Finding a persuasive language of partnership that really 'works' is evidently a pressing priority.

Nor do all groups simply become one big happy family; they can be divided or excluding. This may be at the heart of failure rates among group programmes, not just in effectiveness but in recruitment and dropout. Groups can represent a Faustian bargain if they promote the interests of categories among their members at the expense of others – not least, minorities. Hence more research that includes untypical attenders – men, women from minorities, single parents, those with disabilities or outside heterosexual norms, and the growing army of step-parents – would make a timely contribution.

Appreciating the importance of personal identity, group membership, and interaction is a challenge for both research and practice. In the next section a study that engaged with such questions is introduced.

A study of stakeholders' goals and perspectives, based in the UK

The sample

In order to explore the views of diverse stakeholders, the study was designed to be inclusive both of different parenting programme settings and of different parent identities (Grimshaw and McGuire 1998). Interviews took place with a range of stakeholders associated with three local programmes selected from a national sample of voluntary, 'open access' group programmes. They were meant to represent a variety of geographical areas and potential users. Two were organised in public health service settings catering for young children and the third in a school for 5–11-year-old children. As well as parents, 'agents' – people responsible for funding, coordinating, or delivering programmes or for recruiting parents – were interviewed (Guba and Lincoln 1989).

To obtain a balanced picture, it was essential to contact not only parents who had attended programmes but also parents who had not. Four categories of parent were interviewed: parents who had been on a course and attended most of the sessions (a total of 21 attenders); those who had only attended a small number of sessions (6 drop-outs); those who knew of a course but had decided not to participate (17 refusers); and a further 11 parents who were in effect excluded because they had not been made aware of the programme.

The sampling was designed to include as many social categories as possible. Of the 55 parents in the sample: 71% were women; 78% were white, and the rest came from minority ethnic groups. The most highly represented minority group was African – six in all, including three war refugees. There were individuals from African–Caribbean, Indian, Bangladeshi, and mixed backgrounds.

The majority had a partner, but 9% were parenting alone. Just over half were couples (but were interviewed individually).

Again, a wide range of household incomes were represented in the sample, ranging from less than £100 to over £1000 per week. The largest group (18%) had an income between £300 and £400 per week.

Because views on parenting may be influenced by experiences of stress, a list of stressful situations was constructed by the research team, ranging from the parent's emotional, health, financial, or housing problems to the strains of caring for a large or demanding family. A cumulative stress score was worked out for each parent based on evidence from the interviews. Just over a quarter of parents had no such stresses but the rest had a range of stressful experiences, the majority of whom had up to two stresses.

Views on programmes

How far did the parents in the study regard programmes as relevant to their needs? At what stage would access be useful? How should programmes be delivered? And what should they cover? What would be useful outcomes? The following section explores how far programmes can fit into the agendas of parents themselves, rather than an agenda imposed on them from outside.

Towards the end of the chapter the collective views of those funding, delivering, or recruiting for these particular programmes are compared with parents' ideas.

Consumer information and choice

Despite the attention given to parenting programmes in sections of the press, knowledge about them still seemed restricted. Parents interviewed were asked to identify any programmes for parents which they knew. Apart from basic parent-craft and antenatal classes or post-natal support groups, there was little awareness of parenting programmes.

If partnership-thinking is to advance, attempts to inform parents in general about key features must be accelerated so that they have a reference point from which to assess local initiatives. We would all expect health care initiatives to be publicised; why not parenting services?

Interest in programmes among non-attenders

To overcome the knowledge gap, parents who had no contact with a programme were given some general information and invited to ask questions before their views were sought.

The level of interest which they expressed was relatively high (Table 6.1). A number would have wanted this service in the past but felt that it would not be appropriate now. Others would only want the service if they had a problem or they wanted more specific help. A few were more comfortable with a TV or video presentation.

So what led parents to reject programmes? One attributed her unwillingness to two reasons: strong family support and her resistance to anxiety.

I have never been one for mother and toddlers groups but I have such a large family. I have all that I need and sometimes I do think the mothers and toddlers groups are also for the mothers, you know the contact is there and the worries that they had or . . . I am not a worrier by nature.

Table 6.1 Interest in parenting programmes among non-attenders

Responses	Number
Yes	12
Possibly in past	5
Only if I had a problem	6
No	2
Can't attend	2
Other kind of service	1
TV/Video	2
Total	30

This example illustrates the valuation placed by a parent on support and advice, suggesting that, in this case, this could be obtained within the parent's own milieu, rather than via a programme.

The best stage to attend

Planning the availability of services at times they are needed should take account of parents' preferences. Parents who had attended sessions or expressed an interest in doing so were asked to say when they might wish to take part.

Over half the respondents wished to access a programme before a child reached the age of 3 years. The most popular option was to go on a programme in the child's first year – an idea with a particular appeal to women. Even among the parents with school age children there was a clear preference for an earlier opportunity to attend. Parents saw a programme as a foundation for their careers as parents.

Partnership in the group process

Parents were asked to say what kind of person should be 'a leader'. Instead of simply opting for expertise, they expressed a strong preference for someone who was a parent, or who was both a professional and a parent.

Asked to describe the qualities of a leader, nearly all respondents mentioned qualities such as the ability to communicate and to listen, friendliness, patience, openness, and compassion. The parents clearly wanted a friendly listening partner, as opposed to a didactic teacher. Commenting on how a group had worked in practice, a participant spelled out how the group process translates the messages into something that is more than a distillation of the 'book'.

I think [the facilitator] felt that it's not so much what's in the book that really makes the difference in how things are actually put across, it's how the group as a whole interacts and understands and how much information can be put into it by all the participants, and how it all comes out in the wash basically.

Group membership

Because the group setting is so important, the gender composition of the group can be a major issue for some parents. Most – both men and women – said they would wish their partners to accompany them. However, some were certainly doubtful, feeling that the group discussion would not be so frank or allow feelings to be expressed.

I mean [my husband] went to [a course in baby and infant care] with me but I wouldn't say he learned anything. I think it's somewhere where mums can let go and we can have a moan about the husbands.

Yet fathers' programmes were not favoured. As one father put it:

I just don't think it's in the male make-up to sit there and talk about, I suppose it's interesting for a little while but I don't think blokes tend to click so well.

Evidence from those who attended programmes confirmed the practical importance of acknowledging identities within a group setting.

Some people who did not conform to the typical profile of attenders felt isolated. A sole male attender described how the facilitator's assumptions about her audience pointed up his difference from the group:

a lot of things that she was talking about were all from a female perspective. Obviously she is a woman herself, but they were being aimed at a female audience, and she kept on saying, 'Oh, and Dads', it was almost like 'Oh sorry I forgot you were there.'

For the young refugees the experience of a group reinforced their sense of isolation as foreigners. Even a woman with a different experience of parenting could feel placed on the margin. A mother with a full time job was uncomfortable when home-makers criticised mothers who went out to work.

The context of family and child care

Choices about attendance are affected by family circumstances that structure the parents' attitudes to activities outside the home. Regardless of their preferences about attending with partners, a large majority needed someone to look after the children while they attended a programme. Difficulties with work arrangements were not frequently mentioned. However, for a single parent, cost might be a major deterrent:

the only thing that I do suffer from is babysitters, the young girl down the road costs me £5 each time I have a babysitter. I am not in a financial situation to keep paying out £5 here and there for a baby-sitter.

Hence child care is a primary factor to be considered in developing a partnership with families, especially the most isolated. Such considerations, predictable as they may appear, also help to explain why involving partners in programmes can be troublesome.

Content

The 51 parents with some interest or experience were asked what they wanted to be included in an ideal programme. Fourteen of those who had attended sessions opted for what they had experienced. Seven of the rest went along with what had been described to them. A mother of Asian origin suggested that the normal programme topics were relevant to most parents regardless of background.

Most parents come across, whatever religion or background or whatever, they come across very similar problems, you know, teaching children good behaviour rather than bad behaviour, actively listening to children, what they are saying; these are things you come across whatever language you speak so your . . . sounds fine to me.

In addition, about a quarter of the respondents expressed interest in family and social issues, in child behaviour, and so on. A similar proportion wanted information about child development or health. Fewer – just one in ten – were interested in educational issues for their children. There were several other formulations or suggestions mentioned, such as targeting a particular age group of children. A single parent wanted a course specifically for single parents, endorsing the consideration of individual needs in a group setting.

Views about outcomes

All parents interviewed, whether they had experience of programmes or not, were asked to say what they expected to get out of a programme (Table 6.2). The most frequently mentioned were group outcomes, such as comparing individual experiences with other people's. These were followed, in order of frequency, by a better relationship with the children, greater knowledge, and emotional benefits.

The value of sharing experiences was a frequent theme.

I think if you feel that other parents experience the same problem then it's not just your problem, you are sharing something and it's not just your children that are behaving like that.

Table 6.2 Outcomes envisaged by parents from parenting programmes

Group outcomes e.g. networks friends compare self with others learn from other parents	43 references by 31 respondents
Relationships outcomes e.g. understanding child communication relationship resolve problem less conflict	38 references by 27 respondents
Knowledge outcomes e.g. health outcomes development education	30 references by 25 respondents
Emotional outcomes e.g. less anxiety raise confidence happiness less stress	26 references by 20 respondents

Most importantly, parents were seen as responsible for interpreting the ideas within their own family settings.

You can only go by models. You can't really define everything you've
got to do to be a parent. . . . Children are different; parents are different;
people's circumstances differ. But if you can put them as working
models then you get people thinking.

Parents were then asked to envisage important outcomes for
their *children*. The most frequent replies, from about half the
respondents, mentioned improvements in the parent–child relationship, such as behaviour changes and understanding. Almost
three out of ten referred to a child's emotions, such as happiness
or greater confidence. Only one in ten mentioned particular
aspects of a child's needs, such as being healthy, making educational progress or meeting special needs.

Among policy makers there is a strong wish to identify long-
term benefits from programmes. Parents were asked to think
about 'short-term' and 'long-term' benefits. The short term
meant any benefit occurring immediately or in the months
following a programme. The long term was defined as a period
extending beyond a year after the course.

Parents' sense of the future was not sharply divided into
distinct phases. Many of the responses concerning the short term
were repetitions of previously stated outcomes or combinations
of these. Insofar as it could be recognised, the long term
appeared to be an extension of the present.

However, parents were conscious of the fragility of gains made
during a relatively short programme. Some suggested that they
should be contacted at a later date as a form of auditing progress.
Indeed virtually half the sample said that they would find a
follow-up course useful.

Agents' views about outcomes

In order to compare the outcomes envisaged by the different
stakeholders, similar open ended questions were put to agents. In
Table 6.3, to simplify the comparison, the broad responses about
outcomes were aggregated with responses on the specific outcomes for the short and long term.

Table 6.3 Outcomes envisaged by agents

	Number
For parents	
Emotions such as happiness and confidence	14
Group support	9
Improved relationship with child	7
Personal empowerment	5
Knowledge/understanding	5
For child	
Improvement in child's emotions	3
Improvement in child's behaviour	1
Help with child's identity	1
Improvement in child's social skills	1
Educational progress	2

The consensus of the agents, from various backgrounds, bears interesting resemblances to the views of parents. There was a clear recognition of emotional benefits for parents and for children. This emphasis was particularly evident among facilitators. The enduring supportive functions of the groups were acknowledged.

Parents themselves, I would like to think were more confident, that they are more relaxed and less stressed and that in itself must have a spin off as to how they relate with their children . . . I think the really telling part would be kind of six months down the line, whether they felt that they could, they had sort of kept up some of the resolves and promises they've made to themselves at that time. I think that if the parents actually keep in contact with the programme remain as a support to each other there is more likelihood of that happening.

There was also a feeling that parents should be given the power to shape their own destinies for themselves. The evidence suggests that the service providers shared a broad agenda with parents about the desirable outcomes of parenting programmes. So far, so good. But the idea that partnership is demanding to implement was acknowledged by a comment from one senior coordinator of school-based programmes.

I have a little concern about the word partnership, I am just wondering how much of a partnership there is here, and if again it is basically the school telling the parents what to do . . ., it could be perhaps handled differently, invite them, meet the parents first, to ultimately help them meet their child's needs.

It should be remembered that these service providers were not the authors of published programmes but were committed to delivering services at ground level with no resort to compulsion. Like anyone approaching a market, they had developed a realistic 'take' on the aspirations of their customers for self-realisation in a social context.

Conclusion

Once a dream, flying to the moon became possible when government pressed its resources into action. No one believes that constructing a suite of effective parenting programmes is actually an operational feat comparable to a NASA project. But the 'go-getting' spirit of results-oriented policy thinking can lead researchers and practitioners to focus on the visible engineering of a project, *at the expense of the processes that go on beneath the surface*. These are equally vital to its success. Programmes can be misinterpreted if they are seen purely as pieces of effective hardware. A helpful way of reorienting the discussion about what works is to compare programmes with computing. Hardware is certainly important in providing capacity, ensuring consistency, and maintaining reliability. Nonetheless, running software is *about supplying information and choice to users*. They are attracted to software that addresses them directly, enquires about their needs, links them to like-minded associates, and presents options. It may seem facile to talk about the imperatives of the computer age in a society in which some children fail to have their most basic needs met. However, the efflorescence of personal computing has exploited and revealed one fundamental truth: that *human decisions can be substantially empowered by the promotion of self-activity and self-esteem in a rich, shared information context*.

This UK study has shown that programme organisers are

aware of the significance of such factors. The great need at present is to expand such awareness so that it receives proper attention in the research literature, in planning and in delivery (Lloyd 1999). Partnership can then become more than a marketing slogan and take its place with honour in the lexicon of what truly works.

Acknowledgements

I am grateful to Christine McGuire and Sheila Wolfendale for contributing to my thinking about the implications of partnership and effectiveness. My thanks go to the National Children's Bureau and the Joseph Rowntree Foundation for permission to quote material from the study that promoted these reflections (Grimshaw and McGuire 1998).

References

Barlow, J. (1997). *Systematic review of the effectiveness of parent-training programmes in improving behaviour problems in children aged 3–10 years. A review of the literature on parent-training programmes and child behaviour outcome measures.* Oxford, Health Services Research Unit, Department of Public Health.

Barlow, J. (1998). Parent-training programmes and behaviour problems – findings from a systematic review. In A. Buchanan and B. L. Hudson (eds.), *Parenting, schooling and children's behaviour.* Aldershot, Ashgate.

Dembo, M., Sweitzer, M., and Lauritzen, P. (1985). An evaluation of group parent education: behavioural, PET and Adlerian programmes. *Review of Educational Research,* **55**(2), 155–200.

Dosanjh, J. and Ghuman, P. (1998). Child-rearing practices of two generations of Punjabis: development of personality and independence. *Children and Society,* **12**, 25–37.

Grimshaw, R. and McGuire, C. (1998). *Evaluating parenting programmes: a study of stakeholders' views.* London, National Children's Bureau.

Guba, E. and Lincoln, Y. (1989). *Fourth generation evaluation,* London, Sage.

Halstead, M. (1994). Between two cultures? Muslim children in a Western liberal society, *Children and Society,* **8**(4), 312–26.

Johnson, Z. and Molloy, B. (1995). The community mothers' programme – empowerment of parents by parents. *Children and Society*, **9**, 73–85.

Lloyd, E. (ed.) (1999). *Parenting Matters: what works in parenting education?* London, Barkingside, Barnardo's.

Long, N. (1997). *Parent education/training in the USA: current status and future trends.* Conference on Clinical Child Psychology and Psychiatry at the Royal Society of Medicine. 30 January.

Macdonald, G. and Roberts, H. (1995). *What works in the early years? Effective interventions for children and their families in health, social welfare, education and child protection.* London, Barkingside, Barnardo's.

Medway, F. (1989). Measuring the effectiveness of parent education. In M. Fine (ed.), *The second handbook of parent education.* New York, Academic.

Oakley, A. (1993). *Social support and motherhood: the natural history of a research project.* Oxford, Blackwell.

Samra, B. (1999). Supporting parents through parenting programmes. in S. Wolfendale and H. Einzig (eds.), *Parenting education and support: new perspectives.* London, David Fulton.

Smith, T. (1998). Parents and the community: parents' views and mapping need. In A. Buchanan and B. L. Hudson (eds.) *Parenting, schooling and children's behaviour.* Aldershot, Ashgate, pp. 110–23.

Webster-Stratton, C. and Hammond, M. (1990). Predictors of treatment outcome in parent training for families with conduct problem children. *Behaviour Therapy*, **21**, 319–37.

Webster-Stratton, C. and Herbert, M. (1994). *Troubled families – problem children. Working with parents: a collaborative process.* Chichester, Wiley.

Webster-Stratton, C. and Taylor, T. K. (1998). Adopting and implementing empirically supported interventions: a recipe for success. In A. Buchanan and B. L. Hudson (eds.) *Parenting, schooling and children's behaviour.* Aldershot, Ashgate, pp. 127–60.

7

Do intervention programmes for parents, aimed at improving children's literacy, really work?

Catherine Baillie, Kathy Sylva, and Emma Evans

'We have entered a new century in which learning will define our lives as never before. Whether we succeed and prosper, as individuals or as a country or fail to progress and fall behind, will depend on our knowledge and skills, abilities and understanding.' **David Blunkett (2000), Secretary of State for Education and Employment**

The government is keen to reduce social exclusion by tackling its roots early in childhood through intervention programmes that support parents. There is good evidence that many children who fail to adjust to school by the end of reception year have persisting problems as they grow up. Over time, many become increasingly antisocial and disaffected with school, and underachieve badly. They often require a lot of special educational help and resources. As adults, many end up with few qualifications or skills, and find their lives are unsatisfactory in terms of getting work, and in getting on with people.

In 1997 the Literacy Taskforce argued that parents have a key role in promoting literacy. In this chapter we review the research evidence which supports calls for increased parental involvement in the first years of their children's formal education. We go on to speculate about which elements of intervention programmes aimed at supporting parents to assist their children's reading are necessary for success.

Parental influence on their children's literacy: observational studies

It has long been established that children's reading performance tends to correlate with social class (e.g. Douglas 1964; Kellmer-Pringle *et al.* 1966; Davie *et al.* 1972). Research reported by Hewison and Tizard in 1980, however, seemed to offer a potential means of ameliorating the low performance of working class children. They had found that, within a working class group of children, reading attainment was significantly and reliably related to whether or not children's parents claimed they regularly listened to their children read. About half of the parents of top infants and first-year junior school children that Hewison interviewed said that they regularly heard their children read at home. These children were found to be significantly ahead of other children in reading attainment, even after IQ, social class, and home-background variables had been taken into account.

Other correlational research has since confirmed this observation. Plewis and colleagues (1990) measured the amount of time 6-year-olds in inner London spent in educational activities at home, and found that the activity most highly correlated with reading attainment was time spent reading aloud. An Australian survey of over 5000 primary and junior school children (Rowe 1991) found that reading activity at home (measured as frequency of reading alone, reading to others, discussing reading, and being read to by others) was significantly and positively associated with reading achievement, as well as with the mediating variables of attitudes to reading and attentiveness in the classroom. These associations were stronger than any between socioeconomic status and reading outcomes. The findings of another Australian study (by Share *et al.* 1983) similarly showed that, while indices of socioeconomic status were positively associated with reading performance, specific processes operating within the home (i.e., academic guidance, language models, levels of family literacy, parental participation, and aspirations for the child) were more directly related to student achievement. In their meta-analytic review, Bus and colleagues (1995) found a significant and reliable association between whether parents read story books to their pre-school children and children's reading achievement. The effect size of this association was smaller with older children, presumably because, as children began to learn to read themselves, it was more important whether their parents heard them practice their reading aloud rather than whether their parents read story books to them.

Although these studies demonstrate a clear association between parents hearing their children read and children's reading levels, the association with children's *progress* in school is less clear. Tizard *et al.* (1988) reported that although pre-school advantages in terms of parental help with reading gave children long-term advantage, neither the frequency with which parents heard their children read, nor the frequency with which parents read to their children were related to progress. The results they reported are somewhat confused by the term 'parental help', which in some analyses was limited to parent listening only and in others included behaviours such as talking about books, playing games, flashcards, computer based games, or having books available. Whilst frequency of parent–child reading was not significantly related to progress (i.e. change scores), all other parental behaviours (such as talking about books, playing games) *were* positively related to progress. Tizard *et al.* described their results as 'puzzling and disappointing'.

These studies have demonstrated beyond doubt that many parents (in low and middle class, and black and white populations) hear their children read 'spontaneously'. All of these studies have also found at least some element of spontaneous parental involvement in children's literacy experiences (usually hearing their child read) to be positively related to children's reading attainment. But is the relationship causal?

Parental influence on their children's literacy: Intervention studies

Having established a link between *spontaneous* parental involvement and children's reading attainment, the challenge for research was to establish first, whether parents who infrequently heard their children read could be induced to do so on a regular basis and second, whether this *induced* parental involvement would have similar positive effects on children's literacy and school adjustment.

The Haringey Reading Project (Tizard *et al.* 1982) set out to meet these challenges by (a) introducing a scheme to increase parental involvement in listening to their children read, and (b) using an experimental design to evaluate the effectiveness of this scheme on children's reading attainment. This project ran for two school years, with children from 6 to 8 years, in six consenting schools in a low socioeconomic area. In two schools, one class was randomly selected to receive a parental involvement intervention. In these classes parents were encouraged to hear their children read regularly. Record cards were kept and direct contact with class teachers was made available. There were also repeated researcher visits to children's homes to observe them reading to their parents and to offer advice to parents. At two further schools one class in each school was randomly selected to receive an alternative intervention: that of supplementary teaching in small groups. In scientific terms the Haringey Reading Project had an exemplary experimental design, with within-school controls for the intervention and for alternative treatment groups, and between-school controls for both programmes (as well as an extra two schools with no programme to control for diffusion/contamination effects). However, differences in reading scores for each cohort, and the fact that the ranking of schools was not stable over time, meant that all between-school comparisons were dropped from the final analysis.

At the end of the first and second years of the intervention children in the parental involvement groups were, on average, performing significantly better in reading than the within-school control classes, in both schools. The mean scores for the control classes were in the range which might be expected for a working class sample (Hannon 1987). The mean scores for the parental involvement classes, conversely, were above the national average. The positive effect of parental involvement was evident in groups of children of all abilities, although there is some suggestion that it had a more profound effect on the progress of initially low achieving children (Macleod 1996).

One year after the intervention the preferential effect of parental involvement was only evident in one of the two schools housing this intervention (school 1). Three years after the intervention (by which time the children were 11 years old), the parental-involvement group's level of reading attainment was still significantly higher than the within-school control group's. Hewison (1988) concluded that the parental-involvement intervention had had a lasting benefit. Despite the reported success of the Haringey Reading Project, subsequent studies failed to replicate the results (Ashton *et al.* 1986; Bloom 1987; Hannon 1987).

Hannon (1987) reported a 'replication' of the Haringey study, carried out in Belfield, Rochdale. Hannon's analysis of data from 7-year-old children *before the intervention was introduced* confirmed what had already been established by Hewison and Tizard (1980); that there was a high level of *spontaneous* parental involvement in hearing children read (over half the children were said to read to someone at home at least several times a week), and that frequency of being heard read at home was significantly associated with reading attainment. There was considerable parental involvement in hearing children read before the intervention was introduced. The intervention was simply for teachers to be systematic in encouraging *all* parents to listen to their children regularly, by sending home books and record cards with all children, daily.

Hannon's analysis of adherence to the scheme was encouraging. In parent interviews, all but two children in the intervention cohorts were said to read at least several times a week, and 90% were said to read *almost daily* to someone in the home. Self-reported frequency of reading was confirmed by analysis of reading record cards sent home with books. In terms of reading attainment, however, the results were less encouraging. Although, on average, the project cohorts performed somewhat better on reading tests at the end of the intervention period than pre-project cohorts had done, the difference was slight and not statistically significant.

The Hannon study differed from the Haringey Reading Project in a number of important ways. First, the intervention in the study reported by Hannon was carried out for longer (3 years with children aged from 5 to 8) and, because it was carried out with sequential intake years, class teachers had to participate in, and maintain, the intervention over 5 years. Second, it included only a very limited home visiting component, staffed by class teachers. Hannon believed his study to be superior to the Haringey Reading Project in that the conditions of the intervention were more naturalistic and, therefore, of more relevance to policy. Because the intervention was introduced primarily for educational rather than research purposes, however, the evaluation had to take the form of a cohort comparison. Therefore, what the study gained in ecological validity it lost in scientific credibility.

The problem with the cohort comparison was that there were considerable year-to-year fluctuations in the reading attainments of different pre-project cohorts (mean scores on the NFER Reading Test A ranging from 91.3 to 96.8) and between different project cohorts (ranging from 90.5 to 104.2). Such large fluctuations in mean reading level from one cohort to the next make it impossible to evaluate the efficacy of the parent involvement scheme. Of the six cohorts for which NFER Reading Test A scores were reported, however, only one cohort (a project cohort) achieved a mean score above national norms and at a level comparable with the parent involvement groups in the Haringey Reading Project.

Null findings in the Hannon study might be explained by the fact that considerable parent involvement in reading and well-developed home–school relations existed prior to the project. For a number of years the school had attempted to work closely with parents, involving them in their children's reading, albeit on an ad hoc basis. The intervention was merely to be systematic in their efforts. Macleod argues that a sensible hypothesis, therefore, would have been 'that the group most likely to benefit from the project were those at the tail end of the distribution curve – the low reading achievers', who were statistically less likely to have parents already involved in their reading. Although this hypothesis was not supported to a statistically significant degree, the proportion of children in the lowest ability group (with standardised scores of 84 or less on the NFER Reading Test A) was 14% in the project group as compared with 26% of the pre-project cohort.

The mixed results from the most rigorous intervention programmes suggest two key factors. First, that the parents of many children, especially those with poorly developed language skills, may need guidance in how to listen and respond to their children's reading. And second, that a key element in programme success is parental commitment and attitudinal change. Toomey (1993) summarised it well: 'The widespread practice of schools sending home books for parents to hear their children read does little to help children most at risk of reading failure . . . (however) *parent training* studies have shown how to bring about substantial improvements in poor readers' interest in reading as well as their reading competence.'

Behavioural approaches to parental interventions

We now have effective techniques for helping parents acquire skills in listening to their children read (Hannon 1995). The most successful ones have a behaviourist slant, although tempered by a collaborative approach with parents and schools working as equals. One strategy is called 'Pause, Prompt, Praise'. This method involves training parents to

(1) pause to allow children to self correct;
(2) give prompts, usually based on meaning;
(3) use praise as a reinforcement for correct reading and the child's independent attempts at self-correction.

This strategy has been successfully used to improve the reading attainment of primary aged children experiencing initial reading difficulties (McNaughton *et al.* 1981; McNaughton 1985).

Another well described, and evaluated, strategy is called 'Paired Reading'. The aim of this technique is to support the child's reading in such a way that the focus is removed from errors, and confidence to attempt new reading challenges is encouraged. This is achieved by the two phases employed by the paired reading technique (Pumfrey 1986):

1. Simultaneous reading: the child chooses a book which the parent and child then read aloud together. The child is to make an attempt at every word. When the child does make an error the parent allows a few seconds for the child to repeat themselves correctly without discussing it.

2. Independent reading: when the child feels ready to read alone they will signal to the parent using a pre-arranged sign, the parent will then stop reading. When the child makes an error or stops reading the parent gives the correct response, which is repeated by the child. Simultaneous reading is reverted to until the child signals their readiness for another attempt at independent reading.

Numerous studies using a simple pre- to post-intervention design have demonstrated significant gains in children's reading ability as a result of paired reading (Topping and Lindsay 1992). In the UK, the Kirklees paired reading project is the most cited of these studies (Topping 1986). This project was set up by the local education authority and the technique was taught by an initial lecture followed by the participants practising the technique, and receiving feedback and individual instruction. For the first 6–10 weeks the involvement lasted for five sessions per week, with each session lasting approximately 5–15 minutes. Teachers reported improved levels of confidence in 71% of children, 65% were reported to be more accurate, and 68% were reported to be more fluent. Paired reading was shown to have beneficial effects on reading accuracy and fluency as well as on confidence, motivation, and classroom behaviour (Topping 1986).

More recent studies, using a randomised controlled study design, show consistent results. Overett and Donald (1998) introduced the paired reading technique in an educationally disadvantaged area of South Africa. Prior to the intervention few children reported having more than two books at home and only just over half belonged to a library. The intervention was run in school and consisted of weekly 1-hour sessions for 6 weeks. The sessions were attended by the class teacher, the children, and a parent or other family member. Emphasis was on regular and positive interaction around the paired reading activity. Prior to implementation of the intervention there were no differences between a control group and the group which was to receive the intervention in either reading accuracy or comprehension. The paired reading intervention was shown to significantly improve reading accuracy and comprehension, as well as children's attitude to reading. A UK study compared paired reading with another intervention, described as 'relaxed reading' (Lindsay *et al.* 1985). Both interventions included an introductory lecture followed by either a weekly home visit or telephone call. Both interventions led to above expected improvements in reading accuracy and comprehension, but no differences between the effectiveness of the two interventions were found.

Although the paired reading technique, and other techniques like it, have demonstrated improvements in children's reading attainment, the mechanism through which the outcome of this association occurs is still poorly understood, and until it is understood the outcome of parental involvement programmes will remain unpredictable. The paired reading technique is a specific, well-described intervention. However, there is considerable variation from study to study in both the teaching of the method and the level of parental adherence to it (Elliott 1991). Again, the process has been shown to be a complex one with not just the quality of parental hearing of their child's reading changing. The amount of time parents and children spend involved in reading activities may well increase, particularly for pairs where books and access to libraries is limited, such as Overett and Donald's sample. Attitudes towards reading have also been shown to change, and the amount of contact parents have with schools and teachers is also likely to alter as a result of some parental involvement interventions. Griffiths and Hamilton's (1985) descriptive account of a pilot project establishing PACT (Parents and Children Together) in one junior school in inner city London reported no statistics or hard outcome data but described a change in the attitudes of parents, teachers, and children. Parents were reported to feel that teachers made an effort to answer their needs and, as a result felt closer to the school and its aims: 'The children themselves displayed a growing awareness to the fact of their parents and teachers exchanging information about them and their work and appeared to greatly benefit from this knowledge.' (p. 11)

Hamilton (1987) went on to explain: 'What must finally be evident is that whatever way parents are working, what they are actually doing is increasing their children's motivation, self-esteem and understanding – all the qualities children so often lack, and which are the keys to learning.' (p. 41)

Any one, or a combination, of these factors may be the 'active ingredients' of parental involvement in children's reading.

Ingredients of a successful parental intervention programme

Two key elements to success are (1) giving parents a positive structured way to interact with their children, and (2) increasing their ability to negotiate with teachers. Research in the UK has demonstrated that we now have effective techniques for helping parents early on in the educational process in acquiring a set of skills to help their children read at home (Hannon 1995). The importance of increasing home–school contact is also consistent with the empirical evidence. Hewison (1982) reported that (in her original survey with Jack Tizard) whether mothers attended open days was positively associated with children's reading test scores. In the Haringey Reading Project a significant number of mothers were of ethnic minority groups and non-English speaking. These families are unlikely to have had strong collaborative links with the school prior to the parental involvement intervention. The regular and supportive home-visiting component of the scheme, as well as the 'school-gate conferences' described by Tizard *et al.* (1982) are likely to have provided an essential bridge providing previously isolated parents with a means of access to teachers and vice versa. Conversely, in the Hannon study well developed home–school relations existed prior to the project, and there was only a limited home visiting component to the intervention. Therefore home–school links were unlikely to be changed to a significant degree, which might explain his null findings.

A major element of the Perry/Highscope project's success, in the USA, was the involvement of parents in the programme for their children. This project gave educational input to deprived children before they went to school. The children have now been followed up well into adulthood. By 27 years, more had completed higher levels of schooling, fewer had been in receipt of state benefits (59% versus 80% of children who had not received the programme), and the level of repeat (five or more) arrests was greatly reduced, 7% versus 35% (Schweinhart and Weikart 1993). This is the most thoroughly assessed long-term follow-up of an early educational intervention, and its lessons are particularly relevant as it demonstrated objectively a big reduction in the crime rate. Furthermore, it clearly evinced the link between scholastic and behavioural problems. Children who fail to adjust to school for whatever reasons have persisting problems as they grow up. Scholastic failure is associated with impaired function in other domains, such as poor peer relationships, emotional disturbance, and behaviour problems (Kazdin 1987). So far there are no published programmes in primary school of which we are aware that address both scholastic and behavioural problems together.

Tackling literacy and behavioural difficulties together: a new approach to supporting parents

In 1999 an innovative community-based intervention to support parents in managing the two sets of child difficulties for which they most frequently seek help, namely behaviour and learning (Family Policy Studies Centre 1995) was begun (Scott and Sylva, in progress). Research confirms that these two problem areas are closely related and combine to lead to serious impairment in adulthood if unchanged. Many children with behaviour problems have severe and persistent reading difficulty. Rutter and Yule (1970) found that a third of 10-year-olds exhibiting antisocial behaviour had reading skills more than 2 years behind that expected, even allowing for their IQ.

Without effective intervention, behaviour problems have a high degree of continuity, with 40% of the children becoming delinquent as teenagers (Robins 1978). The adult manifestations are widespread, including alcoholism, drug dependence, and antisocial personality disorder (Robins and Price 1991), antisocial behaviours such as theft, violence, drunk driving, use of illegal drugs, carrying and using weapons (Farrington and West 1981), and relationship difficulties, including a high rate of marital violence, divorce, and abuse of the next generation of children (ibid.). Like behaviour problems, the continuity of early scholastic underachievement to adulthood is strong, with an association with later failure to get any qualification on leaving school, which in turn predisposes to subsequent unemployment (Maughan *et al.* 1985) and receipt of state benefits (Rutter and Giller 1983).

The project introduced here is innovative because it combines elements which address both of these aspects of child development. It aims to help parents provide the emotional and intellectual framework their children need to get the best out of school, by providing parents with techniques for supporting literacy and behaviour management (Webster-Stratton and Herbert 1994). The aims of the intervention are to:

- Increase parents' ability to manage their children's behaviour, and reduce physical punishment;
- Increase parents' involvement in constructive activities with their children, and reduce neglect;
- Increase parents' involvement with school, and encourage them to practise specific techniques to promote reading;
- Reduce child behaviour problems and management difficulties;
- Improve child literacy attainments.

The project uses (a) a parent training package which has been shown to support the parent–child relationship and improve child behaviour, and (b) a proven parent support programme to address child literacy difficulties. In term one, parents are taught and practise techniques to help prepare their child emotionally and socially for learning. These include how to enhance their child's social skills with adults and children, how to improve their child's ability to concentrate and attend during activities and play, how to enable them to become more self-sufficient and constructively in control of situations, and how to develop their child's impulse control and reduce aggressive outbursts. The methods are taught to parents in weekly groups led by a project officer for child social skills. In the term two the programme helps parents develop their child's literacy skills. They learn specific methods to encourage their child to identify written material in the environment as well as in books, and how to foster their child's interest and skills – be it looking at their cereal packet in the morning, the road signs on the way to school, or a book in the evening. The methods are taught using small groups, but also include individual visits to family homes by the project officer, and some literacy workshops for families. In the term three a mixture of literacy and coping skills is taught.

The Department of Health have funded this major project, taking place over two and a half years in six inner city London schools. Schools were selected if they met the inclusion criteria. These were to have two full-sized reception classes per year, to be outside the Education Action Zone, and to be representative of the borough in terms of proportion of pupils eligible for free school meals and the proportion of pupils with special educational needs. During the project six hundred parents of 5-year-old children in these schools will be screened. Approximately 120 families whose children exhibit disruptive and difficult behaviour will be selected, 60 of whom will be offered the intensive intervention, while 60 will be offered an 'occasional advice' intervention. Measures are being taken before and after the intervention and at 1-year follow-up, and the two approaches will be compared.

We anticipate that increasing parental skill should lead to significant improvements for these children, and better their lives in both the short and the longer term. It should also reduce social exclusion. The results of this project will be reported in 2002.

This chapter began with a review of correlation studies showing that parental help with children's literacy is associated with higher reading attainment. It then reviewed intervention studies which report disappointing results when parents are induced to help their children. It concludes by suggesting that parents need specific and sustained guidance on helping their children and that this guidance is most effective when integrated into a systematic programme for helping parents towards more positive parenting through effective management of children's behaviour.

References

Ashton, C. J., Stoney, A. H., and Hannon, P. W. (1986). A reading at home project in a first school. *Support for Learning*, **1**, 43–9.

Bloom, W. (1987). *Partnership with parents in reading.* London, Hodder & Stoughton.

Bus, A. G., van Ijzendoorn, M. H., and Pellegrini, A. D. (1995). Joint book reading makes for success in learning to read: a meta-analysis of intergenerational transmission of literacy. *Review of Educational Research,* **65**(1), 1–21.

Davie, R., Butler, N., and Goldstein, H. (1972). *From birth to seven: a report of the national child development study.* London, Longman (NCB).

Douglas, J. W. B. (1964). *The home and the school: a study of ability and attainment in primary school.* London, MacGibbon and Kee.

Elliott, J. (1991). The learning opportunities afforded to children by parental involvement in reading. Unpublished PhD thesis, University of Leeds.

Family Policy Studies Centre (1995). *Parenting problems – a national survey of parents and parenting problems.* With Dept of Health and Office of Population and Census Surveys. London, FPSC.

Farrington, D. P. and West, D. J. (1981). The Cambridge study in delinquent development. In S. A. Mednick and A. E. Baerts (eds.) *Prospective longitudinal research,* pp. 137–45. Oxford, Oxford University Press.

Griffiths, A. and Hamilton, D. (1985). Parent-teacher cooperation over reading in a junior school. *Early Child Development and Care,* **20**, 5–15.

Hamilton, D. (1987). Working with parents: the key to learning. *Support for Learning,* **2**(3), 37–42.

Hannon, P. (1987). A study of the effects of parental involvement in the teaching of reading on children's reading test performance. *British Journal of Educational Psychology,* **57**, 56–72.

Hannon, P. (1995). *Literacy, home and school: research and practice in teaching literacy with parents.* Bristol, Falmer Press.

Hewison, J. (1982). Parental involvement in the teaching of reading. *Remedial Education,* **17**(4), 156–62.

Hewison, J. (1988). The long term effectiveness of parental involvement in reading: a follow-up to the Haringey reading project. *British Journal of Educational Psychology,* **58**, 184–90.

Hewison, J. and Tizard, J. (1980). Parental involvement and reading attainment. *British Journal of Educational Psychology,* **50**, 209–15.

Kazdin, A. E. (1987). *Conduct disorders in childhood and adolescence.* Developmental Clinical Psychology and Psychiatry, 9. Newbury Park, CA, USA, Sage.

Kellmer-Pringle, M. L., Butler, N. R., and Davie, R. (1966). *11,000 seven-year olds.* London, Longman.

Lindsay, G., Evans, A., and Jones, B. (1985). Paired reading versus relaxed reading: a comparison. *British Journal of Educational Psychology,* **55**, 304–9.

McNaughton, S. (1985). The influence of immediate teacher correction on self-corrections and proficient oral reading. *Journal of Reading Behaviour*, **13**, 367–71.

McNaughton, S., Glynn, T., and Robinson, V. M. (1981). *Parents as remedial tutors*. Wellington, NZ, CER.

Macleod, F. (1996). Does British research support the claims about the benefits of parents hearing their children read regularly at home? A closer look at the evidence from three key studies. *Research Papers in Education*, **11**(2), 173–99.

Maughan, B., Gray, G., and Rutter, M. (1985). Reading retardation and antisocial behaviour: a follow-up into employment. *Journal of Child Psychology and Psychiatry*, **26**, 741–58.

Overett, J. and Donald, D. (1998). Paired reading: effects of a parent involvement programme in a disadvantaged community in South Africa. *British Journal of Educational Psychology*, **68**(3), 347–56.

Plewis, I., Mooney, A., and Creeser, R. (1990). Tie on educational activities at home and educational progress in infant school. *British Journal of Educational Psychology*, **60**, 330–7.

Pumfrey, P. D. (1986). Paired reading: promise and pitfalls. *Educational Research*, **28**(2), 89–94.

Robins, L. N. (1978). Sturdy childhood predictors of adult antisocial behaviour: replications from longitudinal studies. *Psychological Medicine*, **8**, 611–22.

Robins, L. N. and Price, R. K. (1991). Adult disorders predicted by childhood conduct problems: results from the NIMH epidemiologic catchment area project. *Psychiatry*, **54**, 116–32.

Rowe, K. L. (1991). The influence of reading activity at home on students' attitudes towards reading, classroom attentiveness and reading achievement: an application of structural equation modelling. *British Journal of Educational Psychology*, **61**(1), 19–35.

Rutter, M. and Giller, H. (1983). *Juvenile delinquency*. Harmondsworth, Penguin.

Rutter, M. and Yule, W. (1970). Reading retardation and antisocial behaviour: the nature of the association. In M. Rutter, J. Tizard, and K. Whitmore, (eds.), *Education, health and behaviour*, pp. 289–94. London, Heinemann.

Schweinhart, L. J. and Weikart, D. P. (1993). *A summary of significant benefits: the High Scope Perry pre-school study through age 27*. Ypsilanti, MI, High Scope.

Scott, S. and Sylva, K. Enabling parents: supporting specific parenting skills with a community programme. Research in progress. Funded by the Department of Health.

Share, D. L., Jorm, A. F., Maclean, R., *et al.* (1983). Early reading achievement, oral language ability and child's home background. *Australian Psycholoqy* **18**, 75–87.

Tizard, J., Schofield, W. N., and Hewison, J. (1982). Collaboration

160   *Promoting children's emotional well-being*

between teachers and parents in assisting children's reading. *British Journal of Educational Psychology*, **52**, 1–15.

Tizard, B., Blatchford, P., Burke, J., *et al.* (1988). *Young children in school in the inner city*. Hillside, NJ, Erlbaum.

Toomey, D. (1993). Parents hearing their children read: rethinking the lessons of the Haringey project. *Educational Research*, **35**(3), 223–36.

Topping, K. J. (1986). Effective service delivery: training parents as reading tutors. *School Psychology International*, **7**(4), 231–6.

Topping, K. J. and Lindsay, G. (1992). Paired Reading: a review of the literature. *Research Papers in Education*, **7**(3), 1–50.

Webster-Stratton, C. and Herbert, M. (1994). *Troubled families – problem children. Working with parents: a collaborative process*. Chichester, Wiley.

8

Promoting emotional well-being in schools

Jane Wells

'*For almost a dozen years during a formative period of their development, children spend almost as much of their waking life at school as at home. Altogether this works out at some 15,000 hours during which schools and their teachers may have an impact on the development of the children in their care. . .. Schools can do much to foster good behaviour and attainments and even in disadvantaged areas, schools can be a force for the good.*' **Rutter** *et al.* **1979, pp. 1, 205.**

Schools and the well-being of children

Children spend a lot of their lives at school, and it is well-documented, and not surprising, that schools can have a profound impact on many areas of a child's development besides academic attainment (Rutter *et al.* 1979; Sylva 1994). These influences may be positive or negative; for some children school is a place where they are stimulated, valued, and encouraged to achieve their full potential, while for others it is a place of fear, failure, and alienation. As the requirement for schools to demonstrate their academic success becomes more pressing, it is more important than ever not to lose sight of their influence on the health and well-being of their children. The Education Reform Act of 1988 requires schools to support children's spiritual, moral, cultural, mental, and physical development (Jamison *et al.* 1998), but in practice its implementation varies enormously.

The potential for schools to influence children's mental well-being has stimulated a growing body of work by both practitioners and researchers. Many different outcomes relating to children's mental and emotional health have been targeted, using approaches ranging from changes in the school systems or environment and involvement of the wider community, to changes in learning methods or class environment, curriculum-based approaches, and interventions with individual children, their teachers, or parents. The range of interventions has been matched by the variety of the research evaluating their effectiveness. This chapter draws on evidence from a systematic review of controlled evaluations to reach some conclusions about how school based interventions can influence children's mental health.

Mental health and mental health problems

The original positive and holistic definition of health coined by the WHO over 50 years ago (WHO 1946) was updated by the Ottawa Charter, which described health as 'a positive concept, emphasising personal and social resources, as well as physical capabilities' (WHO 1986). These definitions provide a relevant starting point for considering the attributes of mental health. There is much debate over its definition, or even whether it can be defined at all, given that it is to some extent culturally determined. Mental health is a positive attribute which cannot be defined simply as the absence of mental illness, and it has been argued that mental health and mental illness are not opposite ends of a single continuum, but separate entities (Tudor 1996).

Some attempts at defining mental health encompass such positive attributes as appropriate emotional responses, self-respect and a realistic self-concept, the ability to give and receive love and affection, the ability to plan ahead, openness to new ideas, tolerance, satisfaction with simple pleasures, and the ability to handle problems as they arise and adjust to situations that cannot readily be changed (quoted in Tilford *et al.* 1997). Others also include the absence of negative attributes such as an 'abnormal' level of psychological distress and maladaptive behaviour (NHS Health Advisory Service 1995). Tudor underlines its multifaceted nature, identifying mental health as a generic term encompassing six dimensions: affective, behavioural, cognitive, socio-political, spiritual, and physiological.

Emotional intelligence encompasses many positive attributes of mental health: the ability to identify, understand, express, and manage feelings, and to empathise and build positive relationships with others (Goleman 1996). These characteristics are said to be not only the basis not only for emotional health and successful relationships, but also for success in all other areas of life.

It is perhaps easier to identify factors which contribute to mental health than to define mental health itself. The HEA described a framework with three key areas: healthy social, economic, and cultural structures, social support and social inclusion, and inner emotional resilience (Health Education Authority 1997). A widely used model was put forward by the Carter Commission on Mental Health in 1987 (in Albee and Ryan-Finn 1993), which describes the interaction between environmental and social events and individual assets and liabilities that results in a mental health outcome (Leighton and Murphy 1987). Tilford adapted this to show how these influences contribute to positive mental health (Tilford *et al.* 1997):

$$Mental\ health = \frac{coping\ skills\ +\ self\text{-}esteem\ +\ support\ groups}{organic\ factors\ +\ stress\ +\ exploitation}$$

Factors which increase or decrease the risk of mental health disorders have also been identified, and Buchanan has given examples in Chapter 1. As she points out, there is not a clear link between specific risk factors and disorders, and individual resilience varies enormously. Definitions of mental health problems are influenced by their severity, the social context, and the background and biases of the definer (Albee and Ryan-Finn 1993). This partly accounts for the wide variation in population estimates of psychiatrically defined problems (Newton 1988). In childhood, what might be termed mental health problems or disorders often manifest as emotional or behavioural difficulties or disorders (NHS Health Advisory Service 1995). The epidemiology of such problems follows a continuous distribution ranging from unaffected or mildly affected children to those who are severely disabled by their condition, with no clear cut-off between 'normal' and 'abnormal' (Stewart-Brown 1998).

Mental health promotion and prevention

Definitions of health promotion have developed over time, from a focus on health education and individual behaviour to social and environmental changes which enable people to take control of their own health (Rootman *et al.* 1999). Empowerment, with the active participation of individuals, is seen as a key component (WHO 1986). There has been much theoretical debate about the distinction between promoting mental health and preventing mental health disorders. Some see the two as separate activities, while others define prevention as an element of health promotion (Downie *et al.* 1990), promotion as part of prevention, or suggest abandoning prevention altogether (Tudor 1996). In practice, there is often similarity in the content of interventions which aim to promote mental health or prevent mental health problems, even though the focus of the implementers may vary. This chapter uses a broad definition of mental health, and includes interventions which were identified as either promoting mental health or preventing mental health problems, and which could be classified as primary prevention (with individuals or groups in whom problems are not apparent) (Albee and Ryan-Finn 1993) or universal approaches (applied to total populations) (Kellam and Rebok 1992).

Evaluating mental health promotion

However self-evident the benefits of mental health promoting interventions may seem, without evaluation this cannot be demonstrated objectively. Evaluation can also inform choices between different approaches, and confirm that there are no negative effects. It may even be regarded as unethical not to evaluate, as beneficial interventions may be withheld for lack of evidence.

Evaluating mental health promotion, (and indeed other forms of health promotion as well), presents many methodological problems and is the subject of continuing debate (e.g. Speller *et al.* 1997; Stephenson and Imrie 1998). Experimental methods, particularly the randomised controlled trial, are generally accepted as the best for evaluating most health interventions, although recent evidence suggests that non-randomised studies are not necessarily more biased (Britton *et al.* 1998). Randomisation is less appropriate for interventions whose success is influenced by the commitment and involvement of the subjects, as motivation may be reduced by lack of choice (Stewart-Brown 1999). However, if there is no comparison group intervention effects may be erroneously inferred from changes occurring naturally over time, the effect of regression to the mean (Kirkwood 1988), or the effect of testing (Spirito *et al.* 1988).

The method of evaluation depends on the questions to be answered, but also on practical issues such as the time and resources available. Piette *et al.* identify three main types of evaluation of school health promotion: process evaluation of the implementation and the experiences of those involved (which will usually use qualitative methods); evaluation of the impact on intermediate factors such as educational or environmental factors or behaviour; and evaluation of effects on health and well-being outcomes (which usually requires quantitative measures) (Piette *et al.* 1995). In health promotion, it can be as important to know about the implementation and experiences of those involved, as the effect on outcomes.

There is a need for valid, reliable measures of outcomes relating to emotional and mental well-being. Many different outcomes are relevant, including changes in environmental or social influences on mental health, the impact on individual risk or protective factors, and the effects on attributes of mental health. The quality and relevance of the measures used are important in interpreting evaluation findings. With quantitative measures, effectiveness may be defined by a statistically significant change in a score, but the clinical significance of this is often unclear. A combination of methods would have the most to contribute, as advocated by Paulussen, but he concedes that the ideal approach, using multiple data sources, collection methods, and researchers, would in many circumstances be too time-consuming and expensive (Paulussen 1995). The debate over the best method of evaluation is clearly unresolved and needs to continue. Schools are difficult environments in which to conduct research, but valuable results can be produced if evaluators are explicit about the questions they tried to answer, and the methods used.

Systematic review of mental health promotion in schools – methodology

As the body of research evidence on mental health promotion in schools grows, a synthesis of the findings can underpin the evidence base of practice and future research. Systematic reviews attempt to overcome the publication and reviewer biases inherent in 'expert' and other less systematic reviews. The systematic review methodology specifies the questions, interventions and population of interest, the identification and criteria for inclusion of studies in the review, and analysis of their findings (NHS Centre for Reviews and Dissemination 1996). Systematic reviews were originally applied to assessing the effectiveness of health care interventions, and restricted to randomised controlled trials. However, their potential for contributing to knowledge in other areas such as health promotion, and the need to include studies using other methodologies, has more recently been recognised (Black 1996; Speller *et al.* 1997; Clegg *et al.* 1998; Lister-Sharp *et al.* 1999).

The work described in this chapter is drawn from a systematic review which attempted to answer two principal questions:

- Can school based interventions improve children's mental health and emotional well-being?
- Is it possible to identify attributes which are common to successful school based mental health promoting interventions?

The detailed methodology of the review is summarised in Table 8.1. Search terms using broad definitions of mental health and mental health promotion (Table 8.1 *search terms*) were used to search databases of biomedical and social science literature and education and health promotion research. Other sources included reference lists from published studies and reviews, and internet websites. Contact was also made with many practitioners, researchers, organisations, and academic institutes in the

Table 8.1 Systematic review of mental health promotion in schools – summary of methodology

1.1 Search terms	1.2 Inclusion criteria	1.3 Data extracted	1.4 Quality assessment

Mental health outcomes
Self-esteem
Self-concept
Mental health
Behaviour disorder/adjustment
Social behaviour
Assertiveness training/skills
Coping behaviour/skills
Life skills
Interpersonal/relationship/skills
Social competence/adjustment/skills/
  learning/problem-solving
Emotional adjustment/understanding/
  learning/literacy/awareness
Psychological adjustment/education
Stress
Locus of control
Empowerment
Suicide prevention
Violence/anger/aggression/conflict
  prevention/reduction/
  management
 	
These were combined with search
terms identifying interventions which
were implemented with children in
schools
	Population
	All children in school
	Excluded studies which only involved
	  children already identified as having
	  problems
	
	Intervention
	Completely or partly school-based
	Mainly concerned with promoting
	  mental health or preventing
	  psychological or behaviour problems
	Details of intervention described or
	  available elsewhere
	
	Outcomes
	Some aspect of mental health (see
	  search terms)
	Includes at least one affective or
	  behavioural outcome measure
	Details of outcome measures and their
	  validity/reliability described or
	  available elsewhere
	
	Study design
	Includes a comparison group
	Minimum of 20 per group
	Allocation method clear
	
	Language/time period
	English language only
	Time period covered by available
	  databases
		Intervention
		Aims
		Theoretical background
		Population and setting
		Intervention content and delivery
		
		Evaluation
		Design
		Identification, allocation, and
		  characteristics of subjects
		Outcomes measured and timing
		Measure content, reliability, and
		  validity
		Loss to follow-up
		Analysis and statistical tests used
		Results
		Cost information
		Authors' conclusions
		Assessment of study quality
			Examined the following criteria:
			Description of aims and outcomes
			Description of subjects and
			  comparability of groups
			Description of intervention
			Loss to follow-up, and how accounted
			  for
			Description of outcome measures, their
			  validity and reliability
			Analysis and presentation of results

fields of education, health promotion, child health, and child mental health, in an attempt to identify other published and unpublished work.

The review focused on universal interventions with school children who had not been identified as having a problem. The decision to include only studies which had used a comparison group was based on links with other work (Lister-Sharp *et al.* 1999) and a wish to reach conclusions about effects which could be clearly attributed to the interventions. Where a combination of methods was used, the findings would be taken into account. It was recognised that this approach would exclude a large volume of literature which had much to contribute to the understanding of school based mental health promotion, and there was no wish to devalue research which fell outside the review parameters. The explicit review methodology allows judgements to be made of the evidence on which conclusions are based.

Over 7800 papers and publications were identified in the initial searches, and after viewing titles and abstracts, full copies were obtained of 416 which appeared to be either eligible for inclusion (Table 8.1 *inclusion criteria*) or to provide useful background material. Seventy-one eligible studies were identified. Information about the intervention and its evaluation was extracted (Table 8.1 *data extracted*). Criteria for the quality of non-randomised studies have been identified (Downs and Black 1998), and a checklist based on these was used to objectively assess study quality and identify the elements contributing to good or poor quality in each evaluation (Table 8.1 *quality assessment*).

Results – synthesis of study findings

Despite the fact that these interventions had in common the broad goal of improving the mental health of children in schools, there was a remarkable diversity in their aims, content, the approaches used in implementation, the measures used, and the populations studied. This heterogeneity precluded a quantitative synthesis of the study findings. To allow conclusions to be drawn from a narrative synthesis several approaches to classifying the interventions were used, with the aim of identifying common factors which may contribute to success or failure. There is insufficient space here to present the full results, so a summary will be given, and a representative selection of interventions described.

Twenty-nine interventions focused on younger children (age range 5–10), 34 on early adolescence (ages 10–14), six on late adolescence (ages 14–18), and two across the age range. Fifty-eight of the studies were based in the USA and two in Canada; of the remainder, four were from Australia, four from Israel, and one each from Holland, Zimbabwe, and England.

Three dimensions were considered in classifying the interventions: the aims, the content and delivery, and factors associated with implementation (Table 8.2). The principal aim identified by the researchers, for which outcomes had been measured and reported, was used as the basis for classification (Table 8.2 *aims of interventions*), but in practice many aimed to influence other outcomes as well, and these are also considered in assessing effectiveness. The content and delivery of the interventions encompassed a range of cognitive, behavioural, specific skills-training, and environmental approaches (Table 8.2 *content and delivery of the interventions*). Most used a combination and it was usually not possible to identify a single approach principally responsible for the effect of the intervention, so this classification was not feasible. The content and delivery of interventions will be considered in the narrative. Factors involved in the implementation included the setting, individuals involved, duration, and continuity of the intervention (Table 8.2 *implementation of the intervention*).

Some of the problems associated with judging the success of mental health promoting interventions have already been discussed. In the absence of other indicators, a statistically significant improvement in at least one relevant outcome in the intervention group compared to the control group has been used to indicate effectiveness, despite reservations in inferring clinical significance from this. This is considered in the light of evidence from qualitative assessment where this is available, and the quality of the evaluation.

Table 8.2 Classifying the interventions by aims, content and delivery, and implementation

2.1 Aims of the interventions	2.2 Content and delivery of the interventions	2.3 Implementation of the interventions
Promotion Promoting positive affective outcomes which are attributes of positive mental health and/or protective Promoting skills which are protective of mental health Promoting behaviour which reflects or promotes positive mental health **Prevention** Preventing or reducing negative affective ('internalising' problem) outcomes Preventing or reducing negative behavioural ('externalising' problem) outcomes	Didactic instruction, information giving Discussion Modelling based on video, tapes, stories, puppets, teachers, peers Role play, practice with feedback Reward systems Training in relaxation or coping with stress Self-monitoring or diary-keeping Promoting achievement, promoting helping activities Skills training and rehearsal (e.g. social problem-solving, communication, interpersonal skills) Changes in the class or learning environment Changes in school systems or environment	**Setting** Class-based Extending beyond the classroom involving part or all of the school Involving the school and wider community **Individuals involved** Teachers Outsiders (e.g. specialists delivering specific lessons) Significant others (parents or peers) **Duration** Brief (a few days or weeks) Throughout a school term or year Long-term changes **Continuity** Intermittent (e.g. a weekly session) More continuous (e.g. changing the learning environment some or all of the time) Continuous or permanent changes (e.g. in school systems)

Results – aims of the interventions

Fifty-two of the 71 evaluations demonstrated a significant improvement in the affective outcome related to their main aim, using outcome measures for which there was some evidence of reliability and/or validity, and information about the content. Table 8.3 summarises these findings. All but eight of the studies demonstrating effectiveness and three of those demonstrating ineffectiveness were judged to be of good or reasonably good

Table 8.3 Number of studies showing a significant improvement in outcome, classified by the main aim of the intervention

Aim of the intervention	Significant improvement		No significant improvement	
Promoting positive affective outcomes				
Self-esteem/self-concept/self-efficacy	16	(2)	8	
Empathy	1	(1)		
Internal locus of control	2			
Understanding emotions	1			
Promoting protective skills				
Social, communication, SPS skills	14	(4)	2	(2)
Coping, assertiveness, decision making skills	5	(1)	2	(1)
Promoting positive behaviour				
'Adjusted' behaviour	2			
Reducing negative affective outcomes				
Depressive symptoms	1		2	
Anxiety or stress	3		3	
Hopelessness, loneliness, suicide potential	2			
Reducing negative behavioural outcomes				
Problem behaviour	5		2	
Total	52	(8)	19	(3)

Number in brackets denotes number of the total judged to be of poorer quality.

quality. The largest group of interventions aimed to improve self-esteem, self-concept, or self-efficacy. These have been grouped together as they describe related attributes and are often not clearly distinguished in interventions or in the measures used to evaluate them. Many more interventions were principally aimed at positive (health promoting) rather than negative (preventing) outcomes, and a higher proportion of the health promoting interventions were effective, although there was considerable overlap in content.

Results – implementation of the interventions

There was no clear pattern of effectiveness related to the setting and individuals involved in implementation (Table 8.4). Fifty-eight interventions were solely classroom-based, most involving teachers, outsiders, or both. Too few involved parents or peers to allow lessons to be drawn about the relative benefits of these approaches. Few interventions attempted to broaden their implementation beyond the classroom by involving the rest of the school, and only four studies involved the wider community. Examples of programmes in different settings will be described below.

The duration of the interventions ranged from a few days to several years, and many were implemented intermittently while some involved continuous changes. There were 37 intermittent interventions lasting less than 3 months and of these over half had no effect, compared with less than a quarter of the remainder.

The majority of studies did not evaluate long-term outcomes. Five studies evaluated outcomes 6 months or more after completing a brief (less than 3 months) intervention, and only one found any longer-term effect. One medium-term (20 weeks) intervention found some maintenance of effect 1 year later. Three studies evaluated outcomes three or more years after completing an intervention lasting at least a year, and two of these found that benefit was maintained. Ten studies evaluated outcomes in ongoing interventions which had lasted at least 6 months, and all but two found significant benefit.

Table 8.4 Number of studies showing a significant improvement in outcome, classified by the setting and individuals involved in implementation

	Teacher	Outsider	Outsider + teacher	Parent/peers +/- teacher/other	Total
Class-based	13 *7*	20 *5*	6 *2*	4 *1*	43 *15*
Class + part or whole of school	3 *1*			3 *1*	6 *2*
School + community				3 *1*	3 *1*
Total	16 *8*	20 *5*	6 *2*	10 *3*	52 *19* *

* One additional ineffective intervention was conducted in separate sessions by outsiders and peers.
Interventions showing no significant improvement are indicated in italics.

Examples of interventions and evidence of their effectiveness

Findings of some of the better-conducted evaluations will be described, grouped according to the implementation of the intervention.

Interventions involving the school and community

The concept of the Health Promoting School developed during the 1980s from work undertaken by WHO, with the aim of developing schools which enable pupils, teaching and non-teaching staff, parents, and the community they serve to take action for a healthier life, school, and society. The 12 criteria for a health promoting school are grouped into three domains: the school ethos and environment; the curriculum; and links with home, other schools, and the community. The criteria specifically propose the active promotion of the self-esteem of all pupils, and also highlight the importance of the health and the role of staff (Parsons *et al.* 1996).

An evaluation of this approach in English schools compared 13 intervention primary and secondary schools with 26 'reference' schools over 3 years (Jamison *et al.* 1998). The schools were supported by project staff and were allowed up to £18 000 for health promotion initiatives and staff training to address the three domains of the criteria. Activities included the involvement of pupils in school planning and development, school policies on areas of health promotion, and curriculum changes. There was considerable variation in implementation in different schools, so that the input evaluated was in effect the additional funding and support. Outcomes generally improved in all schools over time, but the rate of improvement in self-esteem was greater in some pilot schools. The evaluation includes much qualitative data which supports the value of the approach for teachers and pupils.

The School Development Project was an earlier intervention with a population of mainly African–American, socioeconomically disadvantaged children in New Haven, Connecticut, which changed the school systems and environment and promoted community involvement. The three main elements were a school management team involving both staff and parents, a mental health team which addressed global school climate issues and individual staff and student concerns, and a programme which encouraged parents to participate in planning and decision making in the school. It also included community based projects involving school children, and social activities.

The evaluation compared two intervention schools with two control schools. Haynes found that after 1 year children in the intervention schools had significantly improved self-concept scores, compared with control children (Haynes and Comer *et al.* 1990). Cauce found some evidence of longer-term benefit (although in a less methodologically sound study), with improved self-concept and academic performance in intervention children compared with controls 3 years after the children had left their elementary school (Cauce *et al.* 1987). These studies support the beneficial effect of a 'whole school' and community approach.

Interventions involving the school

The Child Development Project (CDP) was a continuous long-term intervention designed to improve cognitive, affective, and behavioural aspects of children's development, and promote the understanding of and concern for others. The aim was to establish a 'caring classroom environment' by using cooperative and helping activities, positive discipline techniques, role plays, games and stories, and modelling of positive examples of behaviour. The approach was not limited to the classroom but extended to the whole school and also included some community activities. Teachers were trained in a week-long workshop and on a continuing basis throughout the school year, and parents were involved in developing some of the activities. Children entered the programme in kindergarten and continued it throughout elementary school.

In a well designed evaluation in six Californian elementary schools where it had been implemented for a maximum of 4 years, a significant effect was found on children's social problem solving and conflict resolution skills, measured in role-play situations, with improvements increasing over time (Battistich *et al.* 1989).

Another study compared CDP schools with a school using a competitive reward-based system, and no-intervention control schools (Benninga *et al.* 1991). The aim was to compare the effects of the organisation of learning activities and the incentive structure (whether extrinsic using rewards, or intrinsic using perceived relevance) on interpersonal behaviour, interpersonal understanding, and self-esteem. Over 4 years the CDP students had higher intrinsic motivation for prosocial acts, and the reward system students had higher self-esteem, but no significant differences were found on other measures. The mixed results of these two CDP studies mean that it is difficult to draw firm conclusions, although more weight should probably be attached to Battistich's positive findings which are based on a higher quality evaluation.

The Resolving Conflict Creatively Programme (RCCP) started in New York in 1985 with the aim of transforming the culture of schools, to enable them to teach elementary school children non-violent ways of dealing with conflict, and increase their understanding of their own and other cultures. Components include a teacher training course, curriculum-based classroom instruction in creative conflict resolution and assistance in implementation from project consultants, training of selected students to act as peer mediators, and parent training in dealing with conflict.

A large evaluation comparing RCCP with control schools found positive effects on teacher-reported violence, student problem-solving strategies, and self-esteem. Benefits were less in children whose teachers taught fewer RCCP lessons, and in children in high risk classrooms and neighbourhoods (Aber *et al.* 1998). Previous qualitative evaluations reported positive findings from both teachers and students (Metis Associates 1990).

A number of workers have highlighted school transitions as times of particular stress following which children's emotional well-being and school achievement often deteriorate. The School Transition Environmental Project (STEP) attempted to help children between the ages of 11 and 14 cope better when changing school. The environment in the new school was reorganised to increase social stability for these students, and their home-room teachers were given a more central role in administration, counselling, and family links. This intervention was evaluated in two studies (Felner *et al.* 1982; Felner *et al.* 1993). STEP students scored better on measures of self-concept and teacher-rated behaviour over the year following the transition, and also had more positive experiences of the school environment than control students. An assessment after 5 years found that STEP students had lower absenteeism and school dropout. These studies provide some evidence that school environmental changes can improve emotional well-being.

Continuous class-based interventions

Hawkins *et al.* (1991) evaluated a class based intervention based on a model which assumes that prosocial development is facilitated by social bonding, which it aims to promote in families and schools. Teachers were trained in proactive classroom management methods such as the use of praise and encouragement, in interactive teaching methods, and in the use of a cognitive problem-solving curriculum. Seven-week parent training programmes were also offered. The aim was to reduce antisocial behaviour.

The subjects (520 American elementary school children) were evaluated after the intervention had been in place for 2 years. The main outcome assessed was teacher report of children's antisocial and problem behaviours, analysed by gender and race. White boys receiving the intervention were scored as being significantly less aggressive and antisocial, and white girls receiving the intervention scored significantly better on self-destructive behaviour, compared with controls. No benefits were seen in black children. The authors conclude that this was either due to a tendency of the mostly white teachers to rate white children more favourably, or because the intervention was better suited to the cognitive and affective styles of white than black children. The majority of parents did not participate in parent training and the effect of this component is not clear.

This is a promising intervention in focusing on long-term improvements in classroom environment and teacher practices, and there is some evidence that it improved externalising antisocial behaviour in white children. However, this study highlights the difficulty of eliminating bias when outcomes are assessed by individuals who have been involved in the intervention and are unblinded to group allocation.

Intermittent class-based interventions

Learning environment   A number of programmes used cooperative learning techniques, based on the 'Jigsaw classroom' method proposed by Aronson *et al.* which aims to develop a supportive learning environment, promote social competence and peer relationships, reduce individual competition, and ultimately improve academic outcomes (Aronson *et al.* 1978). Students work together in small groups, each member being responsible for teaching part of the curriculum to the rest of the group. A large study in Israel evaluated its effectiveness in improving the social acceptance and self-concept of ethnic minority students. Cooperative learning for 4 hours a week over 12 weeks or a programme of social activities were both found to prevent the decline in social self-concept which occurred in control children (Eitan *et al.* 1992).

Roswal *et al.* found that a group of 7th-grade, mainly African–American students had improved self-concept and reduced tendency to school dropout after a 16-week period of daily sessions of cooperative peer teaching, compared with traditional learning methods (Roswal *et al.* 1995). An evaluation of cooperative learning approaches used 3–4 times a week over a 10-week period with 5th-grade American children found improvements in teacher-rated behaviour but no effect on self-concept, compared with traditional teaching approaches (Wright and Cowen 1985). Another study assessed its impact on self-esteem, locus of control, and attitudes to peers and school when used for 2 hours a week over a school year (Moskowitz *et al.* 1983). Implementation in some classrooms was found to be incomplete, and no beneficial effect on affective outcomes was found, although intervention children had more positive perceptions of the class environment.

Overall, there is limited evidence for the benefits of cooperative learning in promoting children's mental health. The studies with the most positive findings are in particular populations, so although the approach may be promising, the results are not generalisable.

Educational achievement   The Mastery Learning programme was based on the hypothesis that failure to master core tasks would lead to depressive symptoms, and that improving competence in these tasks would reduce them (Kellam *et al.* 1994a). It was implemented with 1st-grade children in 19 urban elementary schools in Baltimore, USA, and used a flexible group based approach to improve reading attainment.

It was evaluated over a period of 6 months using a measure of reading achievement and a depression inventory. At pre-test there was a significant relationship between lower achievement and higher depression score, and the findings at post-test linked a greater gain in achievement with an improvement in depression compared to the pre-test. A high prevalence of depressive symptoms as measured by the scale (which was well-validated) was found, but the clinical significance of this is not clear. This was a large study, and although loss to follow-up was high there is some support for a link between increasing achievement and decreasing depressive symptoms.

Skills training   Many interventions aimed to improve protective skills, either as the main aim or together with other outcomes. Most of these were curriculum-based and a number target various aspects of social skills. One of the commonest approaches is the development of social problem-solving (SPS) skills, because of research which has demonstrated a link between these skills and adjustment (Shure and Spivak 1982), although these findings have not always been replicated. The specific skills encompass problem identification and definition, generating alternative solutions and deciding between them, implementing a solution, and evaluating its effectiveness. They also include the need for self-control, and awareness and understanding of others (Elias and Clabby 1992).

The Rochester SPS skills programme was evaluated in two relatively large studies involving 2nd–4th-grade American children (Weissberg *et al.* 1981a,b). It comprised 52 sessions over 13 weeks implemented by class teachers based on an established curriculum. The syllabus covered identifying feelings, and recognising and solving interpersonal problems using an 8-step process, and used structured lessons with role-play, video modelling, workbooks, games, and discussion. Parents were also offered parent training in one study but few completed it. Post-test improvements were found in some measures of SPS skills and teacher rated behaviour (although both studies were potentially biased). Neither study found any link between SPS skills and behavioural adjustment.

The Rochester curriculum was also evaluated with Australian 7–9-year-olds (Sawyer *et al.* 1997). At 1-year follow-up, intervention children rated their own ability to deal with problem situations significantly higher than controls did. No differences were found in teacher and parent rated behaviour. Two brief interventions aimed at teaching problem solving steps using modelling, discussion, and role-play found short-term improvements in SPS skills (McClure *et al.* 1978; LeCroy and Rose 1986).

A Dutch study aimed to teach the main principles of decision-making to 12–13-year-olds (Taal and Sampaio de Carvalho 1997). It consisted of 9 weekly sessions using discussion and assignments, based on a published programme delivered by class teachers. At post-test the 87 intervention students had significant improvements in the understanding of decision-making concepts, and in locus of control related to achievements and social relations, compared with controls.

A number of assertiveness training programmes aimed to increase affective outcomes such as adjustment and self-esteem (Vogrin and Kassinove 1979; Waksman 1984a,b; Stewart and Lewis 1986). Most were relatively brief and involved a small number of subjects, and results were mixed. Two studies found post-test improvements in self-concept but larger, well-designed studies would be needed to support this finding.

The evaluations of skills-training approaches demonstrate that skills such as social problem-solving can be taught in schools, although only one study provided evidence of longer-term benefit. An associated impact on affective outcomes might be expected but has not been clearly demonstrated in these studies.

Affective outcomes The Promoting Alternative Thinking Strategies (PATHS) programme aims to improve understanding of emotions, promote emotional development, teach social problem-solving skills, and prevent behavioural problems (Greenberg *et al.* 1995). It comprises 60 lessons delivered by teachers throughout the school year, using didactic instruction, role-play, discussion, modelling by teachers and peers, social and self-reinforcement, worksheets, and generalisation techniques, to enable teachers and children to apply the lessons learnt to other aspects of school.

It was evaluated in 192 2nd–3rd-grade American children. Using a standard interview assessing emotional understanding, PATHS children were found to have significantly improved ability to discuss, recognise, and understand their own and others' feelings at post-test compared with control children. This study lacked information on some methodological details but provides fairly good evidence that PATHS improves emotional understanding in addition to the developmental changes which occur over time. This is a promising intervention from which positive effects on other affective outcomes might also be expected, but were not assessed in this evaluation.

The programme evaluated by Schulman *et al.* aimed to directly improve self-esteem and self-concept by using film clips to stimulate discussion of self-concept themes. This was a relatively brief class-based intervention comprising 12 sessions delivered by class teachers using set materials over 6 weeks. The evaluation recruited 886 6–8th-grade students in Chicago schools, with low loss to follow-up, and found significant improvements in self-esteem and academic and social self-concept in experimental children after the intervention (Schulman *et al.* 1973).

Henderson evaluated the 'Toward Affective Development' curriculum, which aimed to develop self-awareness and understanding of feelings and their relationship with interpersonal events, and improve social skills. It consisted of 23 weekly sessions administered by a facilitator, and was evaluated in 231 5th and 6th graders in two suburban American schools, with random allocation of classes to either affective education alone, affective education with parental involvement consisting of a newsletter and seminar, or no-intervention control (Henderson 1987). Both the intervention groups improved significantly in alternative thinking (the ability to generate alternative solutions to interpersonal problems, tested in hypothetical situations), and the group with parental involvement also scored significantly higher on self-esteem. The additional benefit of the parental intervention component is perhaps surprising given its low-key nature.

Two brief interventions aimed to prevent depressive symptoms and depressive 'cases' in a general high school population (age about 15) (Clarke *et al.* 1993). One consisted of three structured lectures about depression, and the second consisted of a lecture followed by four sessions of guided exercises and problem-solving. Both assumed that encouraging students to increase their involvement in pleasant activities would reduce depressive symptoms, and neither had any effect. These were reasonably good quality evaluations which demonstrated clearly that brief didactic interventions were not effective.

Training in relaxation and the use of mental imagery were used in two brief interventions to reduce stress (Zaichkowsky and Zaichkowsky 1984; Stanton 1985). One found a reduction in state anxiety and physiological measures of stress, while the other found improved scores on a stress inventory at post-test and at 6 months. These studies support the potential of relaxation training, but larger more generalisable studies are needed to confirm these results.

A number of studies have evaluated interventions aiming to reduce adolescents' suicide potential. A 12-week curriculum-based programme in Israel covered understanding distress and its responses, developing coping skills, empathy, help-seeking behaviour, and the ability to identify distress in others (Klingman and Hochdorf 1993). It was delivered by school counsellors and psychologists using instruction, discussion, modelling, role-play, and audio-visual and written materials. Experimental students' scores on an index of potential suicide (with items on depression, anxiety, and emotionality), and on knowledge of coping skills, improved significantly after the intervention. Another study, also based in Israel, used 7 weekly 2-hour workshops involving semi-structured discussion covering describing and working through experiences, feelings, and coping (Orbach and Bar-Joseph 1993). Post-tests found a decrease in suicidal tendency in most intervention groups, and an increase in ego identity and coping skills in some. These were large studies, and while both had some methodological flaws there is some support for the immediate beneficial effects of interventions aimed at reducing suicide potential, although there is no evidence on longer-term effects or benefit relative to more generic interventions.

Behaviour   The Good Behavior Game (GBG) is a reward-based intervention which aims to discourage maladaptive (particularly shy and aggressive) behaviour by rewarding teams of children for appropriate behaviour during specified time periods throughout the school week. Two studies evaluated its implementation in Baltimore schools. In Dolan *et al.*'s study, teachers rated the GBG children as having less aggressive behaviour than controls at post-test (Dolan *et al.* 1993). Kellam *et al.*'s study evaluated children who had been involved in the GBG for 2 years, up to 4 years after completion, and found no difference on teacher assessments of shy and aggressive behaviour compared with control groups (Kellam *et al.* 1994b). These were large studies, but both lacked data on the similarity of groups at the start and appear to have relied on unblinded teacher assessments. The evidence on the effectiveness of this reward-based behavioural approach is therefore mixed; it may improve behaviour in the short term but there is no evidence of longer-term impact.

A number of curriculum-based programmes aimed to reduce problem behaviour. One used a photograph and accompanying social scenario together with discussion, role-plays, and conceptual activities to teach impulse control and anger management, and increase empathy (Grossman *et al.* 1997). Class teachers taught it over a 6-month period. The evaluation involved 790 2nd and 3rd grade children in 12 schools. No significant changes in teacher- or parent-reported behaviour were found, but there was some improvement in both negative and positive behaviours in intervention children using a direct observation measure. Unfortunately this measure had only moderate reliability, so although the study was otherwise well designed, this positive finding must be treated with caution.

Two studies evaluated a violence prevention curriculum used with predominantly African–American students aged 11–13 (DuRant *et al.* 1996; Farrell and Meyer 1997). The curriculum covers knowledge about violence, alternatives to violence, and anger management, mainly through lectures and role-play. Orpinas *et al.* evaluated another violence prevention curriculum which also included interpersonal problem-solving (Orpinas *et al.* 1995). All three studies found reductions in self-reported aggressive behaviour immediately after the interventions, but effects were lost at 3-month follow-up.

Conclusions

School-based interventions can have a significant impact on the mental health of the general population of children. The majority of studies included in the review demonstrated a positive impact on a mental health-related outcome. Benefits have been shown in interventions with a wide range of approaches, from changes in systems and environment affecting the whole school and community, to changes in the class environment or teacher behaviour, and intermittent approaches directed at developing specific skills or behaviours, improving achievement, or promoting specific affective outcomes.

The diversity of interventions, and sometimes the absence of information, made it less easy to identify attributes responsible for their success, but there were some common factors. Most of the interventions were relatively brief, intermittent, and class-based approaches, and these were the least likely to be effective. Maintenance of effect was only assessed in a minority of studies, but longer-term benefits were more likely after longer interventions. Approaches aimed at health promoting outcomes were more numerous, and generally more likely to be effective than those with a preventive focus, but there was a great deal of overlap between the two.

There is evidence to support the effectiveness of a multifaceted whole school approach, which may also involve the community, and of environmental changes within the school. There is some limited evidence to support the benefit of changes in teacher behaviour or learning environments, and increasing educational achievement can also improve mental health outcomes. Skills such as social skills can be taught in schools but an associated impact on affective outcomes was not demonstrated conclusively. It is also possible to increase children's understanding of emotions through a classroom intervention. Relaxation training has some potential in reducing stress and anxiety. Interventions aimed at reducing suicide potential, and reward-based or curriculum-based interventions aiming to reduce problem behaviour, both had some immediate impact but long-term effects were not demonstrated.

Implications for future practice and research

This review focuses on universal school-based interventions aimed at improving children's mental health, which were evaluated using a controlled study design. These studies have provided evidence of the effectiveness of many interventions in improving mental well-being, at least in the short term. Given the difficulty of conducting this sort of research in schools, these positive findings are impressive. However, the findings of some of the studies could have been strengthened by giving more information on areas such as the comparability of the groups, details of measures used and complete reporting of outcomes, and information about losses to follow-up. In addition, information about the relative costs and benefits of different interventions is crucial if implementation is being considered, but none of the studies described here included any evaluation of cost or cost-effectiveness. Further debate is also still needed on the methodology of evaluating mental health promotion. Few of the studies described here used a combination of methods, but where they did this provided valuable additional information on areas such as implementation and the experience of the subjects.

Only one UK-based study met the review inclusion criteria. There is much good work going on in schools in the UK, and some controlled studies are in progress, while some has been evaluated using other methodologies. A recent Scottish initiative has compiled an extensive database of programmes aiming to promote children's social competence (University of Dundee 1999). However, as this review demonstrates, a much greater volume of work has come from the USA. Much of this is allied to the Collaborative for the Advancement of Social and Emotional Learning (CASEL), an innovative and wide-ranging initiative which aims to increase awareness, and facilitate implementation and evaluation of educational efforts to promote social and emotional learning in young people (Collaborative for the Advancement of Social and Emotional Learning 1999).

Unfortunately the generalisability of most studies to the UK context cannot be assumed, but lessons can still be drawn about the type of programmes whose implementation might be considered. The Personal Health and Social Education curriculum provides an opportunity to implement the type of session- or curriculum-based intervention found to be effective in some of these studies. While not all have been shown to deliver longer-term benefit, there are clearly some which can, and programmes would need to be carefully chosen and evaluated with this in mind. However, longer term, more integrated approaches seem to offer a better chance of lasting improvements in children's mental well-being. The health promoting schools approach, which addresses the school ethos and environment and the wider community as well as the curriculum, may offer a better chance of contributing to children's positive mental well-being in the longer term than interventions directed at specific outcomes relating to mental health.

At the same time, schools are only a part of children's lives. Some children cannot be reached through school, and the lives of some may be subject to influences much stronger than those they encounter at school. However, it is now well recognised that the responsibilities of schools go beyond teaching and learning, and while school-based approaches should not be regarded as the only answer, they have great potential to contribute to the mental well-being of their children.

Acknowledgements

Katherine Weare of the Health Education Unit, University of Southampton, provided helpful comments on an earlier draft of this chapter.

I would like to thank my colleagues Sarah Stewart-Brown, Jane Barlow, and Jacoby Patterson for help with the systematic review.

References

Aber, L., Jones, S., Brown, J., *et al.* (1998). Resolving conflict creatively: evaluating the developmental effects of a school-based violence prevention program in neighborhood and classroom context. *Development and Psychopathology,* **10**(2), 187–213.

Albee, G, W. and Ryan-Finn, K. D. (1993). An overview of primary prevention. *Journal of Counselling and Development,* **72**, 115–23.

Aronson, E., Blaney, N., Stephan, C., *et al.* (1978). *The jigsaw classroom.* Newbury Park, California, Sage.

Battistich, V., Solomon, D., Watson, M., *et al.* (1989). Effects of an elementary school program to enhance prosocial behavior on children's cognitive-social problem-solving skills and strategies. *Journal of Applied and Developmental Psychology,* **10**, 147–69.

Benninga, J. S., Tracz, S. M., Sparks, R. K., *et al.* (1991). Effects of two contrasting school task and incentive structures on children's social development. *Elementary-School-Journal,* **92**(2), 149–67.

Black, N. (1996). Why we need observational studies to evaluate the effectiveness of health care. *British Medical Journal,* **312**, 1215–18.

Britton, A., McKee, M., Black, N., *et al.* (1998). Choosing between randomised and non-randomised studies: a systematic review. *Health Technology Assessment,* **2**, 13.

Cauce, A. M., Comer, J. P., and Schwartz, D. (1987). Long term effects of a systems-oriented school prevention program. *American Journal of Orthopsychiatry,* **57**(1), 127–31.

Clarke, G. N., Hawkins, W., Murphy, M., and Sheeber, L. (1993). School-based primary prevention of depressive symptomatology in adolescents: findings from two studies. *Journal of Adolescent Research,* **8**(2), 183–204.

Clegg, A. J., Delaney, F., Gilbody, S. M., *et al.* (1998). Undertaking a systematic review: identifying effective interventions in mental health promotion. *Psychiatric Care,* **52**(2), 57–61.

Collaborative for the Advancement of Social and Emotional Learning (accessed 17 Oct. 1999). Web page: http://www.casel.org/

Dolan, L., Kellam, S., Hendricks Brown, C., *et al.* (1993). The short-term impact of two classroom-based preventive interventions on aggressive and shy behaviors and poor achievement. *Journal of Applied and Developmental Psychology*, **14**, 317–45.

Downie, R., Fyfe, C., and Tannahill, A. (1990). *Health promotion models and values*. Oxford, Oxford University Press.

Downs, S. H. and Black, N. (1998). The feasibility of creating a check-list for the assessment of the methodological quality both of ran-domised and non-randomised studies of health care interventions. *Journal of Epidemiology and Community Health*, **52**, 377–84.

DuRant, R. H., Treiber, F., Getts, A., *et al.* (1996). Comparison of two violence prevention curricula for middle school adolescents. *Journal of Adolescent Health*, **19**(2), 111–17.

Eitan, T., Amir, Y., and Rich, Y. (1992). Social and academic treat-ments in mixed-ethnic classes and change in student self-concept. *British Journal of Educational Psychology*, **62**, 364–74.

Elias, M. and Clabby, J. (1992). *Building social problem-solving skills*. San Francisco, Jossey-Bass.

Farrell, A. D. and Meyer, A. L. (1997). The effectiveness of a school-based curriculum for reducing violence among urban sixth-grade students. *American Journal of Public Health*, **87**(6), 979–84.

Felner, R., Ginter, M., and Primavera, J. (1982). Primary prevention during school transitions: social support and environmental structure. *American Journal of Community Psychology*, **10**(3), 277–90.

Felner, R., Brand, S., Adan, A., *et al.* (1993). Restructuring the ecology of the school as an approach to prevention during school transitions: longitudinal follow-ups and extensions of the school transitional environment project (STEP). *Prevention and Human Services*, **10**(2), 103–36.

Goleman, D. (1996). *Emotional intelligence*. London, Bloomsbury.

Greenberg, M., Kusche, C., Cook, E., and Quamma, J. (1995). Promoting emotional competence in school-aged children: the effects of the PATHS curriculum. *Development and Psychology*, **7**, 117–36.

Grossman, D. C., Neckerman, H. J., Koepsell, T. D., *et al.* (1997). Effectiveness of a violence prevention curriculum among children in elementary school. A randomized controlled trial. *Journal of American Medical Association*, **277**(2), 1605–11.

Hawkins, J. D., von Cleve, E., and Catalano, R. F. (1991). Reducing early childhood aggression: results of a primary prevention program. *Journal of the American Academy of Child and Adolescent Psychiatry*, **30**(2), 208–17.

Haynes, N. M. and Comer, J. P. (1990). The effects of a school develop-ment program on self-concept. *Yale Journal of Biological Medicine*. **63**(4), 275–83.

Health Education Authority (1997). *Mental health promotion: a quality framework*. London, Health Education Authority.

Henderson, P. A. (1987). Effects of planned parental involvement in affective education. *School Counselor*, **35**(1), 22–7.

Jamison, J., Ashby, P., Hamilton, K., *et al.* (1998). *The health promoting school. Final report of the ENHPS evaluation project in England*. London, Health Education Authority.

Kellam, S. G. and Rebok, G. W. (1992). Building developmental and etiological theory through epidemiologically based preventive intervention trials. In J. McCord and R. Tremblay (eds.), *Preventing antisocial behavior*. New York, Guilford, p. 170.

Kellam, S. G., Rebok, G. W., Mayer, L. S., and Ialongo, N. (1994a). Depressive symptoms over first grade and their response to a developmental epidemiologically based preventive trial aimed at improving achievement. *Development and Psychopathology*. **6**(3), 463–81.

Kellam, S. G., Rebok, G. W., Ialongo, N., and Mayer, L. S. (1994b). The course and malleability of aggressive behavior from early first grade into middle school: results of a developmental epidemiologically-based preventive trial. *Journal of Child Psychology and Psychiatry*, **35**(2), 259–81.

Kirkwood, B. R. (1988). *Essentials of medical statistics*. Oxford, Blackwell.

Klingman, A. and Hochdorf, Z. (1993). Coping with distress and self harm: the impact of a primary prevention program among adolescents. *Journal of Adolescence*, **16**(2), 121–40.

LeCroy, C. W. and Rose, S. D. (1986). Evaluation of preventive interventions for enhancing social competence in adolescents. *Social Work Research and Abstracts*, **22**(2), 8–16.

Leighton, A. H. and Murphy, J. M. (1987). Primary prevention of psychiatric disorders. *Acta Psychiatrica Scandinavia*, Suppl. 337, Vol. 76.

Lister-Sharp, D., Stewart-Brown, S., Sowden, A., *et al.* (1999). *Health promoting schools and health promotion in schools: two systematic reviews*. Health Technology Assessment, 3, 22.

McClure, L. F., Chinsky, J. M., and Larcen, S. W. (1978). Enhancing social problem-solving performance in an elementary school setting. *Journal of Educational Psychology*, **70**(4), 504–13.

Metis Associates (1990). The resolving conflict creatively program 1988–89: a summary of significant findings. New York, Metis Associates.

Moskowitz, J. M., Malvin, J. H., Schaeffer, G. A., and Schaps, E. (1983). Evaluation of a co-operative learning strategy. *American Educational Research Journal*, **20**(4), 687–96.

Newton, J. (1988). *Preventing mental illness*. London, Routledge and Kegan Paul.

NHS Centre for Reviews and Dissemination (1996). *Undertaking systematic reviews of research on effectiveness*. York, University of York.

NHS Health Advisory Service (1995). *Child and adolescent mental health services*. London, HMSO.

Orbach, I. and Bar-Joseph, H. (1993). The impact of a suicide prevention program for adolescents on suicidal tendencies, hopelessness, ego identity, and coping. *Suicide and Life-Threatening Behavior*, **23**(2), 120–9.

Orpinas, P., Parcel, G. S., McAlister, A., and Frankowski, R. (1995). Violence prevention in middle schools: a pilot evaluation. *Journal of Adolescent Health*, **17**(6), 360–71.

Parsons, C., Stears, D., and Thomas, C. (1996). The health promoting school in Europe: conceptualising and evaluating the change. *Health Education Journal*, **55**, 311–21.

Paulussen, T. (1995). Review of the methodology of school health education evaluation. In D. Piette and V. Rasmussen (eds.), *Towards an evaluation of the European Network of Health Promoting Schools (the EVA project)*. Brussels, Universite Libre de Bruxelles. Section IIB.

Piette, D., Tudor-Smith, C., Rivett, D., and Ziglio, E. (1995). Evaluation, subsidiarity and quality in the European network of health promoting schools. In D. Piette and V. Rasmussen (eds.), *Towards an evaluation of the European Network of Health Promoting Schools (the EVA project)*. Brussels: Universite Libre de Bruxelles. Section IB.

Rootman, I., Goodstadt, M., Potvin, L., and Springet, J. (2000). A framework for health promotion evaluation. In WHO-EURO working group on health promotion evaluation (eds.), *Evaluation in health promotion: principles and perspectives*. Copenhagen, WHO.

Roswal, G. M., Mims, A. A., Evans, M. D., *et al.* (1995). Effects of collaborative peer tutoring on urban seventh graders. *Journal of Educational Research*, **88**(5), 275–9.

Rutter, M., Maughan, B., Mortimore, P., and Ouston, J. (1979). *Fifteen thousand hours: secondary schools and their effects on children*. London, Open Books.

Sawyer, M. G., Macmullin, C., Graetz, B., *et al.* (1997). Social skills training for primary school children: a 1-year follow-up study. *Journal of Paediatrics and Child Health*, **33**(5), 378–83.

Schulman, J. L., Ford, R. C., and Busk P. (1973). A classroom program to improve self-concept. *Psychology in the Schools*, **10**(4), 481–7.

Shure, M. and Spivak, G. (1982). Interpersonal problem-solving in young children: a cognitive approach to prevention. *American Journal of Community Psychology*, **10**(3), 341–56.

Speller, V., Learmonth, A., and Harrison, D. (1997). The search for evidence of effective health promotion. *British Medical Journal*, **315**, 361–3.

Spirito, A., Overholser, J., Ashworth, S., *et al.* (1988). Evaluation of a suicide awareness curriculum for high school students. *Journal of the American Academy of Child and Adolescent Psychiatry*, **27**(6), 705–11.

Stanton, H. E. (1985). The reduction of children's school-related stress. *Australian Psychologist*, **20**(2), 171–6.

Stephenson, J. and Imrie, J. (1998). Why do we need randomised control trials to assess behavioural interventions? *British Medical Journal*, **316**, 611–13.

Stewart, C. G. and Lewis, W. A. (1986). Effects of assertiveness training on the self-esteem of black high school students. *Journal of Counseling and Development*, **64**(10), 638–41.

Stewart-Brown, S. (1998). Public health implications of childhood behaviour problems and parenting programmes. In A. Buchanan and B. L. Hudson (eds.), *Parenting, schooling and children's behaviour*, Aldershot, Ashgate, pp. 21–33.

Stewart-Brown, S. (2000). Evaluating health promotion in schools: reflections from the UK. In WHO-EURO working group on health promotion evaluation (eds.), *Evaluation in health promotion: principles and perspectives*. Copenhagen, WHO.

Sylva, K. (1994). School influences on children's development. *Journal of Child Psychology and Psychiatry*, **35**(1), 135–70.

Taal, M. and Sampaio de Carvalho, F. (1997). Stimulating adolescents' decision-making. *Journal of Adolescence*, **20**(2), 223–6.

Tilford, S., Delaney, F., and Vogels, M. (1997). *Effectiveness of mental health promotion interventions: a review*. London, Health Education Authority.

Tudor, K. (1996). *Mental health promotion: paradigms and practice*. London, Routledge.

University of Dundee (accessed 17 Oct. 1999). *Promoting social competence*. Web page: http://www.dundee.ac.uk/psychology.prosoc.htm/.

Vogrin, D. and Kassinove, H. (1979). Effects of behavior rehearsal, audiotaped observation, and intelligence on assertiveness and adjustment in third-grade children. *Psychology in the Schools*, **16**(3), 422–9.

Waksman, S. A. (1984a). Assertion training with adolescents. *Adolescence*, **19**(7), 123–30.

Waksman, S. A. (1984b). A controlled evaluation of assertion training with adolescents. *Adolescence*, **19**(74), 277–82.

Weissberg, R. P., Gesten, E., Rapkin, B., *et al.* (1981a) Evaluation of a social-problem-solving training program for suburban and inner-city third-grade children. *Journal of Consulting and Clinical Psychology*, **49**(2), 251–61.

Weissberg, R. P., Gesten, E., Carnrike, C., *et al.* (19981b). Social problem-solving skills training: a competence-building intervention with second- to fourth-grade children. *American Journal of Community Psychology*, **9**(4), 411–23.

World Health Organisation (1946). *Constitution*. New York, WHO.

World Health Organisation (1986). *Ottawa charter for health promotion*. Ottawa, WHO.

Wright, S. and Cowen, E. L. (1985). The effects of peer-teaching on student perceptions of class environment, adjustment and academic performance. *American Journal of Community Psychology*, **13**(4), 417–31.

Zaichkowsky, L. B. and Zaichkowsky, L. D. (1984). The effects of a school-based relaxation training program on fourth grade children. *Journal of Clinical Child Psychology*, **13**(1), 81–5.

9

Making and implementing timely legal decisions for children: research on a court sample

Joan Hunt

'In any proceedings in which any question with respect to the upbringing of a child arises, the court shall have regard to the general principle that any delay in determining the question is likely to prejudice the welfare of the child.' Children Act 1989, Section 1(2)

Introduction: the issue of delay

Children who need the protection of the state because of deficits in parental care are already seriously disadvantaged (Bebbington and Miles 1989). It is therefore vital that state intervention does not further prejudice their life chances. The likely harmful effects of delayed decision-making in court proceedings about children was recognised for the first time in UK legislation in the Children Act 1989.

The principle enacted in the legislation, that delay was potentially damaging and should be avoided, was informed both by a venerable general literature on attachment and separation (Bowlby 1971; Rutter 1972; Wolkind and Rutter 1973) and more specifically, by studies on children in public care and those who had been abused. In 1973, for example, Rowe and Lambert published their seminal study, *Children who wait*. This highlighted the numbers of young children who were 'drifting' in long-term public care because there was little active planning for their future although there was no real chance of rehabilitation. Lynch and Roberts (1982), in their follow-up study of abused and neglected children, showed that those who did well were less likely to have experienced protracted proceedings. The importance of early decision-making was reinforced by a series of studies on outcomes for children admitted to public care (Department of Health 1991). Jones emphasised that children cannot wait – although abusive families can change they may not be able to do so in time to meet their children's developmental needs (Jones 1987, p. 410). At a conference organised to highlight the importance of preventing delay the courts were urged to take into account the differences between a child's and an adult's sense of time, the impact of delay on attachment and security, and the indirect effects of uncertainty in the child's carers (Socio-Legal Centre 1992).

The Children Act, however, also embodies another potentially conflicting imperative, that wherever possible children should be maintained within their own families of origin without the use of compulsory intervention (Department of Health 1989). This, too, was based on substantial research evidence which indicated the need for caution in separating children from their families: research, for instance, on the uncertainties and disadvantages of public care (Rowe 1985; Stein and Carey 1986; Heath *et al.* 1989); or a raft of studies commissioned by the Department of Health (Rowe 1985) suggesting that compulsory intervention was being overused and did not result in better planning for children. Research in progress under a later Department of Health programme, (subsequently summarised in Child Protection, Messages from Research, Department of Health 1995) was also reporting that too many children were being drawn into the child protection system unnecessarily and that local authorities needed to 'refocus' their efforts towards supporting families.

Thus the decision of whether and when to invoke the legal process in protecting children has become an even more difficult balancing exercise under the Children Act than it was hitherto, while once proceedings have begun the requirement to make decisions as quickly as possible has to be weighed against the need to make the best possible decision. The possibility that the legal processes and social services set up to protect children may inadvertently further jeopardise their well-being is an uncomfortable one for those who daily labour with the complexities of safeguarding children. The research findings presented in this chapter, however, demonstrate that there are serious grounds for concern about delay in making and implementing decisions for children before, during, and after court proceedings, and that changes in policy, practice, and the legal framework are needed if the welfare of children is to be more effectively promoted.

The research studies

The two studies whose findings are reported here were part of a large programme of research commissioned by the Department of Health to evaluate the operation of the Children Act 1989. The first project – *Statutory intervention in child protection, the impact of the Children Act 1989* – was designed to evaluate the effect of the Act on the use of legal intervention in child protection cases and the management of proceedings by the courts. The research took place within three predominantly urban local authorities, with racially and ethnically mixed populations. It included cases heard at all levels of court within three court circuits.

There were two phases to the research, spanning implementation of the new legislation in 1991. The pre-Children Act phase, a retrospective analysis of court and Social Services files, covered 104 child protection cases in which the local authority applied for compulsory powers in care, wardship, or matrimonial proceedings in 1989–90. The second phase looked in detail at 83 cases in which care proceedings, the only route now available to the local authority, were initiated in 1991–93. In addition to documentary evidence, the post-Act research also involved observation of court hearings and interviews with adult family members and a range of practitioners – lawyers, social workers, guardians *ad litem* (specialist social workers appointed by the court in England and Wales to safeguard and represent the interests of children) and members of the professional and lay judiciary. The final report of this research was submitted to the Department of Health in 1996 and subsequently published as *The last resort: child protection, the courts and the 1989 Children Act* (Hunt *et al.* 1999).

The second study – *Outcomes of judicial decisions in child protection cases* – followed up 131 of the 133 children involved in these proceedings 2–4 years after the final hearing, through analysis of Social Services files, interviews with adult family members and practitioners, and a postal survey of guardians *ad litem*, lawyers, and social workers. This research report was submitted to the Department of Health in 1998 and published as *The best-laid plans* (Hunt and Macleod 1999).

Looking back: from intervention to outcome

At the point fieldwork was completed on the *Outcomes* project, 105 of the 131 children appeared to be permanently placed, having either been rehabilitated with their birth families, or settled into a substitute placement. On average, by the time permanency was achieved, almost 3 years had elapsed from the point Social Services had become continuously involved. For almost a quarter this interval exceeded 4 years, with durations for some particularly unfortunate children being as long as 7, 8, and 11 years. Moreover, for many children, concerns had been expressed about their welfare well before the start of the period of continuous involvement which eventually led to court action, the average interval being almost 4 years, with a third ranging between 4 and 15 years. Of particular interest are the 34 children whose eventual destination was substitute care and whose welfare had given continuous concern since infancy. On average, by the time these children's futures were settled, they were between 3 and 4 years old, the oldest being 8.

One in six children, however, were in an even worse plight in that, two or more years after the end of the court proceedings, their future was still uncertain, either because they had never been placed, or placements had broken down. Social Services had been continuously involved with these children for an average of 6 years, with the futures of individual children in limbo up to 7, 8, or even 10 years later.

As indicated earlier, the Children Act lays a duty on the *court* to avoid delay in children's cases. Analysis of the 25 sample cases in which it had taken more than 4 years of continuous welfare involvement to achieve permanency, however, revealed that even where court proceedings were very lengthy, these were never the most time-consuming part of the process. Thus the research showed that while there could be no room for complacency within the family justice system, the focus of attention needed to broaden substantially to take in the wider picture. Making timely decisions for children, it was concluded, has to become a more central objective of the child welfare system before and after as well as during court proceedings.

Delay in invoking the court process

Most children subject to care proceedings come from families already enmeshed in the child protection system. Four in five of the sample cases were active immediately prior to the events precipitating proceedings; three in five had been continuously worked with for at least the previous year, the mean per authority ranging from 17 months to over 3 years. In half the cases at least one child was already on the Child Protection Register while in a quarter there had been previous serious consideration of court proceedings .

Comparison of the cases reaching court before and after the Children Act revealed a consistent picture: after the Act, legal proceedings were even less likely to be an early response to child abuse or neglect. A higher proportion of the post-Act cases were already being worked with prior to the decision to take court action; they had been worked with for longer; more services had been provided. It was also evident that the voluntary approach was more likely to be persisted with in the face of difficulties: the children had been on the Child Protection Register for longer, there were more cases where services had been refused, where children were being looked after by the local authority, where court action had been previously considered. It seemed clear that the Children Act had achieved its objective of making local authorities think hard before bringing proceedings (Department of Health 1989). Such success, however, had its downside, as interviews with practitioners revealed:

When do you say enough is enough? You create a supportive, very comprehensive package, you put in a lot of resources and nothing happens. Do you go through it all again? I agree you need to demonstrate it's been done but someone somewhere along the line needs to say we've done as much as we can. (Social worker, 1994)

What I do have anxiety about is the delay imposed by local authorities on themselves – the resources they throw at families in an attempt to engage the court machinery are in my view entirely misplaced and extremely dangerous for the children. Because when they finally come to court they are horribly damaged. (Judge 1995)

Reservations about the length of time it took to institute proceedings were expressed by at least one practitioner in 27 of the Children Act cases, to which the researchers would add another seven. This amounts to two in five cases, rising to seven in ten of those in which proceedings were brought in order to place the children in permanent substitute homes. One such case was that of Marie, aged eight by the time proceedings were started.

Marie had been accommodated (in state care on a voluntary basis) for 6 months. Her mother suffered from a long-term psychiatric illness and Social Services had been working with the family for years, providing respite care on numerous occasions. By the time Marie was accommodated for the last time she was displaying signs of serious disturbance. As the guardian *ad litem's* report said:

The work done with this family has been extensive. Social work time, practical resources, in-home support, additional professional consultation and direct work have all been attempted in various combination. The professional and practical resources of the Health Authority and Education Department have also been extensively deployed.

If I have a criticism it is that all the help being offered may have obscured the Department's capacity to think about the repetitive nature of events, i.e. to stand back and think about this child's position in her family. Workers have been understandably sympathetic to mother herself, but this too may have resulted in the child's needs being neglected.

There is now sound research evidence that parental compliance with support and services does not predict future success. . . . Mother follows a high risk pattern. Children in such families are very likely to be seriously deprived of any sense of permanency in childhood. The long term damage caused in such families is well documented. . . . I appreciate that in situations where there is neglect it is difficult to judge when parenting slides over into not being 'good enough'. That point arose for Marie some time before she was accommodated.

Marie's period in accommodation was used constructively and decision-making was impressively tight. Unfortunately that was not always the case: delay and drift were evident in the case of many accommodated children. There appeared to be four main factors: tardy social work decision-making in the absence of a clear timetable; reluctance to accept lack of progress with reha-bilitation plans; anticipated difficulties in satisfying the statutory criteria where the parents were not threatening removal; and delays in implementing decisions by local authority legal depart-ments.

Throughout, the fact that the children were no longer at risk of significant harm from poor parental care meant that any sense of urgency had usually dissipated. On average, the 21 accommodated children in the sample had been looked after for almost 9 months, while five had been away from home for periods ranging from 12 to 18 months. Yet most of them were very young, almost all under a year at the point they became accommodated. Another 6 months, on average, would elapse before the court made a final decision while those facing a future outside their kinship networks – at least half – would have to contend with further delay and at least one more set of court proceedings before their future was legally secured.

Reducing pre-court delays

Children subject to care proceedings, of course, represent only a fraction of child protection cases, which are typically managed on a voluntary basis (Department of Health 1995). In seeking to promote the welfare of the majority, by pursuing a legitimate, even laudable, policy of maintaining children in their families of origin wherever possible, it has to be acknowledged that it may not be possible altogether to avoid compromising the welfare of the rest.

However, the research did suggest ways in which decision-making in these very difficult cases might be improved. The

Children Act has undoubtedly sharpened the dilemmas intrinsic to child protection work and the importance of professional judgement cannot be over-emphasised. It was concluded that practitioners needed more training in assessment skills generally, and in the requirements of the legal process in particular. Case recording needed to be more structured and systematic, using running summaries, regularly updated chronologies, and periodic assessments of the child's needs and the extent to which those needs are being and can be met within the family. Under current practice 'taking stock' often seemed to occur only when there was a change of worker, information could be lost, and it might only be in the process of compiling statements for court that the full picture became clear, or even that the case files were read. The *Framework for the assessment of children in need and their families*, (Department of Health 2000), is thus a very welcome development. Given good quality supervision/consultation and time for practitioners to reflect as well as act, all unfortunately too often in short supply, considerable improvements in decision-making might be anticipated.

Better assessment, however, is not the whole story. The research suggested that minimising delay requires some attitudinal change, in particular acknowledging the limits of voluntary intervention and the value, in appropriate cases, of compulsion. Research into both these topics is urgently required. Social workers need a better understanding of the legal framework, and greater confidence and competence in operating within a legal forum. Key to this is making greater and earlier use of the expertise of local authority legal departments so that social work and legal thinking proceed in tandem.

Ultimately, the remedy may lie in the establishment of a different type of court system for family cases, more akin to the French model where there does not appear to be such a gulf between courts and welfare agencies. (Cooper *et al.* 1995) Within the current structure, however, it was suggested that a new discrete order, under which short-term interventions could be authorised, might offer a strategy for action in cases where workers currently feel immobilised by the constraints of the law, allowing for the development of a more constructive relationship between the judicial and welfare domains.

Delays within the court process

Improvements in assessment and decision-making processes might be expected to speed up the court process since the number of inadequately prepared cases reaching court should decrease. One of the striking findings of the research was the high proportion of cases (two-thirds) in which proceedings were started before the local authority had decided what they would be seeking at the end of the day. Thus it was only in a minority of cases that the court was being asked to act in a traditional way – that is, giving a decision on the basis of evidence. Typically the purpose of proceedings was to provide a legally protected space in which solutions could be worked out and, usually, assessments undertaken.

The appeal courts have ruled that 'purposeful' delay is legitimate (C v Solihull Metropolitan Borough Council [1993] 1FLR 290 at 304) and trumps the principle of the avoidance of delay. It is hard to gainsay the argument that the objective is to reach the best outcome for the child as quickly as possible, not to make any decision so long as it speedy. From the child's point of view, however, precious time is still passing without any guarantee that 'purposeful delay' will in fact be of any benefit, not simply a blind alley which only postpones the point at which decisions can be made. However, although courts may be extremely dubious of the value of further enquiry, it was apparent in the research that they are generally reluctant to refuse leave. Empirical evidence on the outcomes of assessments in the course of court proceedings is thus very much needed to inform the difficult balancing exercise the court has to carry out.

It would be misleading, nevertheless, to suggest that if only the local authority could get its act together the problem of delay in the court process would disappear. Thirty-nine reasons for delay during proceedings were identified in the sample cases and most cases were affected by more than one, the average being four, with one case experiencing eleven. In order to examine the association between sources of delay and case duration these factors were grouped into six broad categories (purposeful delay (2 in 3 cases); changes in the configuration of the case (1 in 3); parallel court proceedings (2 in 5); family non-cooperation

(2 in 5); resource difficulties (2 in 5), and miscellaneous disruptions (2 in 5)). Analysis revealed that delay arising from resource problems (lack of court time, problems in obtaining expert reports, funding, or places for assessment) had the greatest impact on case duration, adding, on average, 14 weeks to the length of proceedings.

Practitioner interviews confirmed these findings. Although a wide range of factors were identified as causing delay there was a remarkable consensus on the major problems: assessments, experts, and above all, lack of court time, particularly in the higher courts. Over and over again the same diagnosis was proffered:

All these discussions about delay relate to court time. Yes of course the question of delay had to be addressed but they should have done that by providing more court time. If they're not going to do that they may as well not open their mouths. That's probably not absolutely the answer and in some cases there clearly was unacceptable delay due to lack of organisation on the part of the local authority and lack of push on the part of parents' solicitors. And maybe those sorts of delay have been reduced by the Act. But every day what we face is the problem of not being able to get cases heard because there is no court time and that is the great frustration. (Solicitor)

Speeding up the court process

Reducing delay in the court process, a key objective of the Children Act (Mackay 1989), has also been one of its most signal failures (Bracewell 1995; Hale 1995; Hunt 1996). Only one in ten of the sample cases completed within 12 weeks, the time frame to which courts were originally encouraged to work (Children Act Advisory Committee 1992), the remainder taking twice (38 cases) three times (12) or even four times (5) as long, with a mean duration of 18 weeks in the Family Proceedings Court and 30 in the county court. Nationally collected statistics showed that the problems were even greater elsewhere in the country, the average duration of cases completing in 1994 in the county court, for instance, being 37 weeks, rising to 44 weeks in the High Court (Children Act Advisory Committee 1993–94).

Legislative good intentions have not been without impact. The pre-Act phase of the research showed that proceedings at each court level had been even slower. Considerable headway has been made in re-framing delay as a problem to be addressed rather than tolerated; case management by the court, the central strategy in the prevention of delay, has been accepted and is seen to provide a means of keeping both courts and practitioners 'on their toes' and preventing cases 'going to sleep'. These are considerable achievements. What else could be done?

Increasing resources for family work, particularly in relation to court time and the supply of experts, and deploying existing resources more effectively, are obvious solutions. It is impossible to avoid the conclusion that the system is simply inadequately resourced to meet the Act's laudable objectives. Case management is as yet both an imperfectly developed art and one which is inconsistently applied. Nor, despite this being a radical departure from traditional court practices, has there been any systematic evaluation of its effectiveness and there has been little dissemination of good practice. Locally based strategies to identify and address sources of delay are needed: while the factors which can cause delay are universal, the extent to which they do so will vary according to local circumstances. As mentioned earlier, greater realism and robustness may be needed in considering requests for assessments in individual cases – how much information is really needed to make a well-founded decision? In some cases, as a recent court judgement has emphasised (Re D and K (Care Plan: Twin Track Planning) (1999) *The Times*, 29 July) twin-tracking may need to replace sequential planning so that where the original plan does not work proceedings are not delayed by the lack of a contingency plan.

Finally, it was apparent that some cases are held overly long in the court system because the Children Act prevents courts imposing conditions on the use of care orders or reviewing their implementation. While the research so far available (Social Services Inspectorate 1998; Hunt and Macleod 1999; Harwin and Owen, in progress) does not bear out the suspicions which have been voiced about the implementation of care plans (Thorpe and Clarke 1998), measures to increase court confidence, including some restrictions on local authority discretion and the institution of feedback mechanisms would, it is argued, be beneficial and could result in shorter proceedings.

Delays in implementing court decisions

Restoring to courts the right of review the High Court enjoyed in wardship proceedings prior to the Children Act might also help to prevent post-proceedings delay in the implementation of court decisions. For while there was no evidence of local authorities wilfully disregarding the plans worked out in the care proceedings, the *Outcomes* study demonstrated that there was legitimate cause for concern about the speed with which those plans are actioned. Delay was evident in: clarifying initial plans; implementing initial plans; recognising the failure/non-feasibility of the initial plan; making and implementing new plans; legal planning and legal processes.

Harwin and Owen's (in press) research suggests that it has become unusual for final orders to be made, particularly care orders, while the plan for the child remains undecided. Proceedings in 11 of the sample cases in this earlier research, however, ended while a range of options were still being explored: adoption or long-term foster care (4 children); public or kinship care (3); rehabilitation to the birth family or substitute care (3). On average it took 4 months to resolve the uncertainties while one unfortunate child, whose care proceedings had already lasted for 16 months, remained in limbo for a further 15 while fruitless attempts were made to find a relative willing to care.

Firm intentions in themselves, however, were no guarantee of speedy implementation, even when the need for urgency was clear. Ben was already 7 years old when a care order was made and, unusually, his mother had agreed the adoption plan. Given Ben's age and level of disturbance the need for expedition was repeatedly stressed in the care proceedings. However, after a brief flurry of activity the momentum dissipated and it was not until Ben was transferred to a worker in a long-term team, 18 months later, that the process was resurrected.

Ben's case was undoubtedly one of the worst examples of preplacement drift and there were some cases in which plans were implemented with commendable speed. More than half the placements envisaged in plans put to the court were made within 6 months. However, around one in four took more than 12 months to achieve and one in five more than 18, lending weight to practitioner perceptions that:

The local authority seem to heave a sigh of relief when the order is obtained and neglect to follow through. (Guardian *ad litem*)

We whack them through to care orders and then they just sit around. (Local authority solicitor)

There's too much focus on child protection, too little on the long term. Everyone is rushing around to rescue the child from a risky situation then quite suddenly it becomes unimportant. (Team manager)

It was also noticeable that even where the plan was unequivocally for substitute care it was comparatively unusual for much to be done to progress that plan while the court proceedings were still ongoing and only one case where an application was made for a freeing order alongside the care order.

At the point the research concluded there were 49 children in the sample whose initial placement plans had either not been achieved (14) or had failed (35). In about a third of these delay was evident in either abandoning the initial plan or implementing a new one.

When care proceedings on Joseph (aged two) and his sister Molly (six) ended they were living with their mother in a residential placement. Eight months later the family returned to the community, despite a number of incidents of abuse, worrying in their nature if minor in terms of physical injuries. Over the next 18 months, despite an intensive and comprehensive support package with which the mother entirely cooperated, the assaults continued and there was evidence from the children's increasingly disturbed behaviour that they were suffering emotional harm. However, it was not until a major incident occurred that the children were removed. Both children were accommodated while a specialist assessment was made, which concluded, 10 months later, that a permanent substitute family was needed. By this time Molly was nine, Joseph was five, and care proceedings had once again been instituted.

Reducing post-proceedings delay

With the exception of tardiness in terminating some parental placements, it was clear from the research that the greatest problems arose in cases where the plan was for long-term substitute care. Delay and drift in the management of the placement finding process were apparent in almost every case where the plan was for long-term foster care, while among children who were to be placed for adoption there was not a single case in which there was no evidence of delay in either local authority or legal processes. The research report to the Department of Health therefore put forward a number of ideas to tackle this lamentable state of affairs. Despite considerable practitioner support for a system of court review, it was not considered that this was the most important requirement. What was far more important, it was argued, was to encourage and enable local authorities to put their house in good order. The following recommendations were made.

- Care orders should not be made while there is significant uncertainty about the future, and should be supported with firm, clear, and as far as possible detailed care plans which specify how, by whom, and over what timescale the plan will be implemented, and confirm that any resource implications have been authorised at an appropriate departmental level.
- As far as possible preparations for placements in substitute care should begin before proceedings are concluded.
- Information systems should be established capable of tracking the progress of cases, monitoring the implementation of plans, evaluating their outcome, and identifying reasons for failure.
- A designated senior officer should be charged with specific responsibility for overseeing the implementation of plans.
- A substantial element of independent scrutiny should be built into the reviewing process for children being looked after.
- Services should be structured to provide for more effective liaison and mutual understanding between child protection and family placement services.
- Systems should be established to ensure that legal and social work planning proceeds in tandem.

- There should be a substantial increase in resource for services for looked-after children.

Recent Department of Health initiatives aimed at improving local authority services for children – for instance *Quality Protects* – the government's £375 million programme 'for transforming the management and delivery of children's services' (Department of Health 1999) and guidance on care plans (Department of Health 1998) are thus very much to be welcomed. Innovative approaches such as concurrent planning (Katz 1990), now being piloted in the UK by the Manchester Adoption Society and evaluated by researchers funded by the Department of Health, are also very positive steps forward. They suggest that one of the fundamental principles of the Children Act, that decision-making for children needs to be timely as well as sound, may at last move beyond the realm of rhetoric, at least within the welfare system as it operates either side of court proceedings. It is now time, therefore, for the spotlight to turn again on the period of the court proceedings themselves, to evaluate the efficacy of the delay-reduction strategies which have now been operating for almost a decade with apparently no more than partial success, and to think harder about how the legal process might be made to work more effectively to promote the well-being of children.

References

Bebbington, A. and Miles, J. (1989). The background of children who enter local authority care. *British Journal of Social Work*, **19, 5**.

Bowlby, J. (1971). *Attachment and loss*. Penguin, London.

Bracewell, Mrs Justice (1995). Comment. *Family Law*, 25 February, 55.

Children Act Advisory Committee Annual Reports, 1992, 1993–94. Lord Chancellor's Department.

Cooper, A., Hetherington, R., Baistow, K., *et al.* (1995). *Positive child protection: a view from abroad*. Lyme Regis, Russell House.

Department of Health (1989). *An introduction to the Children Act*, London, HMSO.

Department of Health (1991). *Patterns and outcomes in child placement*. London, HMSO.

Department of Health (1995). *Child protection: messages from research*. London, HMSO.

Department of Health (1998). *Quality protects: framework for action*, London, Department of Health. (Available from DH Distribution Centre, PO Box 410, Wetherby LS23 7LN.)

Department of Health (2000). *Framework for the assessment of children in need and their families.* Department of Health.

Hale, Mrs Justice (1995). Foreword. In R. White, P. Carr, and N. Lowe (eds.), *The Children Act in practice*, p. v. Butterworths.

Harwin, J. and Owen, M. (in progress). *The Implementation of care plans.*

Heath, A., Colton, M., and Aldgate, J. (1989). The education of children in and out of care. *British Journal of Social Work*, **19**, 447–60.

Hunt, J. (1996). Care proceedings under the Children Act: the continuing problem of delay. *Childright*, September, **129**, 12–14.

Hunt, J. and Macleod, A. (1999). *The best-laid plans: outcomes of judicial decisions in child protection proceedings.* London, The Stationery Office.

Hunt, J., Macleod, A., and Thomas, C. (1999). *The last resort: child protection, the courts and the 1989 Children Act.* London, The Stationery Office.

Jones, D. P. H. (1987). The untreatable family. *Child Abuse and Neglect*, **11**, 409–20.

Katz, L. (1990). Effective permanency planning for children in foster care. *Social Work*, **35**, 3.

Lynch, M. A. and Roberts, J. (1982). *Consequences of child abuse.* Academic, London.

Mackay of Clashfern, Lord, L. C. (1989). *HL Official Report.* 5th series, clause 720.

Rowe, J. and Lambert, L. (1973). *Children who wait.* London, Association of British Adoption Agencies.

Rowe, J. (1985). Social Work Decisions in Child Care – Recent Research Findings and their Implications. London. HMSO.

Rutter, M. (1972). *Maternal deprivation re-assessed.* Penguin, London.

Social Services Inspectorate (1998). *Care planning and court orders: monitoring the Children Act 1989 – court order study.* London, Department of Health.

Socio-Legal Centre for Family Studies (1992). Avoidable delay in child care proceedings. Conference Report. Papers presented by J. Harris-Hendricks and D. Glaser: The psychiatric view. Bristol, Socio-Legal Centre for Family Studies, University of Bristol.

Stein, M. and Carey, K. (1986). *Leaving care.* Oxford, Blackwell.

Thorpe, Lord Justice, and Clarke, E. (1998). *Divided duties: care planning for children within the family justice system.* Bristol, Family Law.

Wolkind, S. and Rutter, M. (1973). Children who have been in care – an epidemiological study. *Journal of Child Psychology and Psychiatry* **14**(2), 97–105.

10

Improving children's long-term well-being by preventing antisocial behaviour

Deborah M. Capaldi and J. Mark Eddy

'The longitudinal research evidence suggests that antisocial behavior, particularly when some estimate of severity is taken into account, is the single most powerful predictor of later adjustment problems of any childhood behavior studied.' **(Kohlberg *et al.* 1984, p. 132)**

Antisocial behaviour in childhood (e.g. failure to comply with adult requests, aggression toward peers, and stealing) frequently is not a temporary developmental phase, but prognostic of problems which will continue in adolescence and adulthood. In the Oregon Youth Study (OYS), early adolescent antisocial behaviour predicted a wide variety of adjustment problems in late adolescence and early adulthood, including substance use, a poor relationship with parents, rejection by normal peers, association with deviant peers, poor educational outcome, unemployment, arrests, driver's licence suspensions, and early fatherhood (Capaldi and Stoolmiller 1999). Each of these outcomes is related to other failures that can strongly affect not only the individual, but also their friends, family, co-workers, and subsequent children. Given these links, understanding and preventing childhood antisocial behaviour could have long-term benefits in improving the well-being of children, adults, and families. In this chapter, we discuss both basic and preventive intervention research on childhood antisocial behaviour that has been conducted at the Oregon Social Learning Center (OSLC).

Coercion theory: model development and testing

The OYS was designed to test and expand a social learning theory of the aetiology of antisocial behaviour. According to the coercion model (Patterson 1982), the central social process in the early development of persistent antisocial and criminal behaviour is the basic training of children's aggressive behaviour within the family. The primary mechanism for this training is hypothesised to be negative reinforcement. Negative reinforcement of a child's aggressive behaviour occurs when the parent makes a request, the child responds negatively, and the parent backs down (e.g. the parent asks the child to turn the television off, the child yells no, and the parent leaves them watching the television). Through the day-to-day repetition of this process, a child learns that a non-compliant and even aggressive response to a parent can help them get their own way (e.g. not having to turn the television off).

Parents further foster the development of interpersonally aggressive behaviours when they fail to use consistent and effective discipline in response to the child's misbehaviour (Patterson 1986; Patterson *et al.* 1992). Inconsistent discipline may result in a failure to learn impulse control. As Tremblay *et al.* (1999) note, most children have used physical aggression by the end of their second year after birth, and most have either desisted or use less physical aggression by school entry. Failure to use consistent discipline, and exacerbation of and training in aggression through family coercion may result in young children failing to show such developmental improvement. In addition to inconsistent discipline, other parenting behaviours that are associated with conduct problems in children are lack of monitoring or supervision (Stoolmiller 1994), lack of positive involvement with the child (Capaldi and Patterson 1991; Patterson *et al.* 1992), and poor family problem solving (Forgatch and Patterson 1989). Characteristics of the child, such as an irritable temperament or hyperactive behaviour, which make them more difficult to handle, may place them at higher risk for coercive interactions with their parents and for harsh and inconsistent discipline.

Aggressive behaviours learned at home tend to be employed in other key settings, such as school (Ramsey *et al.* 1990;

Stoolmiller *et al.* 1995), where aggressive children are likely to be rejected by prosocial peers and teachers and to have difficulty with academic performance (Dishion *et al.* 1991; DeBaryshe *et al.* 1993). Rejection by prosocial peers effectively cuts a child off from the socialising influence of skilled peers and tends to increase the chance that a child will associate with other aggressive children. Unfortunately, association with other troublesome children tends to reinforce aggressive behaviour and also provide a child with a training ground for yet a new set of problem behaviours (e.g. stealing, vandalism, early drug use).

Contextual factors within the coercion model

All families operate within a larger context of factors that affect internal family process, either in a supportive or detrimental fashion. Such contextual factors include employment changes (Freeman 1983), divorce and parental transitions (Hetherington *et al.* 1981; Capaldi and Patterson 1991; Cherlin *et al.* 1991; Forgatch *et al.* 1996), stress, depression (Forgatch *et al.* 1988; Snyder 1991), parental antisocial behaviour (Farrington 1979), disorganised and high-crime neighbourhoods (Rutter and Giller 1983; Offord *et al.* 1991), and occupation and education (i.e. socioeconomic status (SES); Elliott *et al.* 1985).

Although investigators might agree that both family and contextual factors are significant for child development, there is little consensus about how these variables fit together in determining key outcomes. We posit that many of the effects of contextual variables on antisocial behaviour are mediated through family and peer process variables (Fig. 10.1). Each of the contextual variables shown in Fig. 10.1 has been shown to be associated with antisocial outcomes, and many studies have also demonstrated a mediational relation between context and outcomes. In each case, the mediational process involved either problematic family or deviant-peer group interactions.

Two different processes may account for the association between stable and trait-like versus state-change contextual factors and boys' antisocial behaviour. Contextual factors such as SES and antisocial personality have been found in many studies to be relatively stable characteristics of parents. Both of

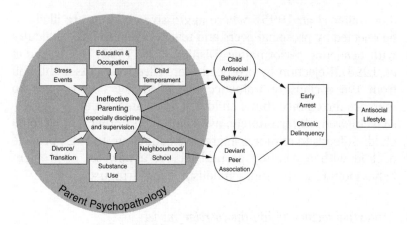

Fig. 10.1 The mediational family model.

these contextual factors have been found to be related to poor child adjustment. These stable contextual factors identify some parents who are at risk because they never learned parenting skills and/or learned some inappropriate parenting behaviours (e.g. harsh and abusive discipline). On the other hand, less stable state characteristics (e.g. stress and depression) are hypothesised to disrupt and diminish parenting by taking the parents' time and attention from their child, or by increasing inconsistent parental responses to the child due to depressed or irritable mood states. The state characteristics are often related to the more stable parental characteristics; thus, their independent causal role may be questionable. Chronic family problems (e.g. parent antisocial behaviour) have been found to predict both family stress and poor child adjustment (Gersten *et al.* 1977; Cohen *et al.* 1987). Thus, in Fig. 10.1 parent psychopathology is shown to underlie both other contextual factors that impinge on the family and poor parenting practices.

As shown in Fig. 10.1, poor parenting practices are associated with the emergence of antisocial behaviour in childhood and also with deviant-peer association (Dishion *et al.* 1991; Patterson *et al.* 1991). It is also hypothesised that there is a direct relationship between child temperament and childhood antisocial behaviour, as well as a direct relationship between neighbourhood factors and deviant-peer association. Adolescents in neighbourhoods and schools with a high deviant-peer density are more likely to become involved with both antisocial peers and delinquency. For example, Wilson (1987) found that, controlling for SES, youth in cities needed more monitoring than youth in the suburbs to prevent them from engaging in delinquent acts. Reiss (1986) argued that in disorganised, high-crime neighbourhoods, parental authority and control is replaced by that of peers, and strong peer-control systems tend to create antisocial subcultures.

The Oregon Youth Study

The OYS comprises a longitudinal sample of two subjects who were recruited by inviting all fourth-grade boys (ages 9–10 years) attending public schools within the higher-crime areas of a medium-sized metropolitan region in the Pacific Northwest of the USA to participate. Of the 277 eligible families, 206 agreed to participate. The sample was representative of the area in being predominantly white (90%), approximately 75% lower and working class, and highly mobile. By age 18 years, 55% of the boys had a police arrest record, and 20% had five or more arrests. Fifty-two percent graduated from high school with their class, and 9% entered a 4-year college. Yearly retention has been 97% or higher through the most recent complete assessment (ages 22–23 years). Recruitment and retention strategies are described by Capaldi *et al.* (1997).

Assessment strategy

Reliable assessment of the day-to-day social interactions that shape child development was central to addressing the hypotheses of the OYS. This was especially crucial in preparing for future intervention studies, as social interactions such as with parents and peers are viewed as more malleable than factors such as child temperament and socioeconomic background. For an assessment of child functioning to be ecologically valid, it must encompass the major social fields in the life of a child, as well as the major interactants. Parents, teachers, and peers are natural raters for the family, classroom, and peer-group social fields, respectively. Such raters are aware of the behavioural standards considered acceptable in their social setting. As the judgements of any given rater tend to be biased to some degree (Patterson and Forgatch 1995), it also is important to collect observational data on a child's behaviour, including his or her interactions with others.

Assessments conducted for all studies at the OSLC include the collection of information via multiple methods, in multiple settings, and from multiple agents. In the OYS, methods included observational assessment of moment-to-moment behaviours as well as more traditional reported data including questionnaires and interviews. In addition, records-based assessment such as court records and school records were collected when appropriate. Settings included the home, the school, and the peer group. Agents included the child himself, parents, peers, and teachers, as well as project staff. Once responses from each individual of interest had been recorded, items were combined into scales (e.g. mother report of son's antisocial behaviour) according to predetermined reliability criteria. These scales and observational measures were then separate indicators of the construct of interest (e.g. antisocial behaviour). Items and scales were standardised as necessary so that the indicator scores, usually averages, were meaningful. For some analysis purposes, taking a mean of the indicators to form a construct score was appropriate. In structural equation modelling, the indicators are considered observed measures of the latent (i.e. unobservable) constructs. Within such models, the estimates of the relations between constructs (e.g. discipline and child antisocial behaviour) tend to be less biased by measurement error.

Testing the coercion model

Hypotheses generated from Patterson's coercion model were tested with the OYS data set. Indicators for parental discipline included observed ineffectual nattering and harsh discipline, as well as ratings and reports of inconsistency and ineffectiveness of discipline. Parents and children reported on supervision, or the monitoring, of the child's whereabouts and behaviour. The antisocial behaviour construct included parent, teacher, child, and peer reports. As reported by Patterson *et al.* (1992), the coercion model was supported for the OYS study. Forgatch (1991) demonstrated that the model generalised to two additional risk samples. The models explained from 30% to 52% of the variance in antisocial behaviour.

Expanding the coercion model

The interrelationship of contextual factors   The various contextual factors depicted in Fig. 10.1 as affecting the family and child are interrelated. For example, experiencing divorce and relationship transitions is related to stress and income. The importance of considering the relation between contextual factors when hypothesising causal associations can be seen in the study of the association between divorce and troubled behaviour in children (e.g. Hetherington *et al.* 1979, 1981; Wallerstein and Kelly 1980). Early research in this area focused on the risk status of the single-parent versus the two-parent family, and the effect on the parents and child of the stress and disruption of the divorce. The entry of a stepfather into the family was thought to decrease antisocial behaviour, at least for boys (Santrock 1972; Tooliatos and Lindholm 1980; Hetherington *et al.* 1981).

Capaldi and Patterson (1991) posited that children's adjustment would be related to the number of parental transitions that had been experienced by the family since the child's birth (0 = intact families with two biological parents, 1 = first separation, 2 = stepfather, 3 or more = second separation, second stepfather, etc.). They tested the association between the boys' risk for poor overall adjustment at Grade 4, and the number of transitions experienced by his parents. Adjustment was the mean of seven constructs; namely, antisocial behaviour, substance use, deviant-peer association, peer rejection, poor academic skills, depression, and low self-esteem. The association between adjustment and number of parental transitions was linear and strong, even after controlling for SES and income. Boys from families who had experienced multiple transitions showed the highest risk for poor adjustment, at 0.5 standard deviations above the sample mean (70th percentile).

Further, it was predicted that parents' antisocial and unskilled behaviour put them at risk for marital transitions *and* poor parenting skills. As expected, mothers' antisocial behaviour was significantly related to the number of marital transitions they had experienced, as well as to poor supervision and participation in fewer activities with their sons. These poor parental practices were, in turn, related to their sons' overall adjustment level (as assessed by the seven constructs described above). There was no direct prediction from number of parental transitions to parenting practices once accounting for parental antisocial behaviour.

Aggression toward partner

An area that has received increased attention in recent years is that of domestic violence, and a major research question regards the role that processes in the family of origin have to play in such behaviour. A fully prospective model of the association of couple's aggression to family-of-origin process has been tested on the OYS sample (Capaldi and Clark 1998). The intergenerational transmission paradigm has predominated in explanations of spousal violence for almost 20 years. However, tests of intergenerational models have been weak because there are virtually no published studies in which aggression between the parents and other family-of-origin variables were assessed during childhood, and then the child's subsequent aggression toward a partner assessed in adulthood. A further weakness is that there has been little specification of the mechanisms or mediational processes that may be involved. The mechanism generally assumed to account for the association between parental dyadic aggression and the boy's later aggression to partner is modelling. It was predicted for the OYS that this commonly hypothesised model would fit the data. However, this model does not include the important construct of parenting practices or the mediating factor of the development of antisocial behaviour. It was hypothesised that unskilled parenting would show a stronger association with boys' antisocial behaviour and, through that, with boys' later aggression toward a partner than would parental dyadic aggression. The association of parental dyadic aggression to the sons' later aggression toward a partner was hypothesised to be due mainly to the fact that antisocial parents are at risk both for aggressive relationships with their spouse and for unskilled parenting practices. Results of the full hypothesised and prospective model are shown in Fig. 10.2 (Capaldi and Clark 1998).

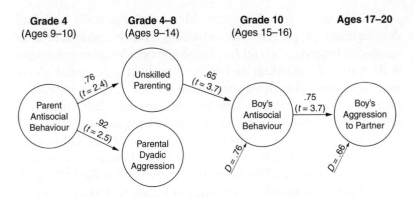

Fig. 10.2   The mediated intergenerational model.

Stronger evidence was found for a mediated pathway via unskilled parenting and boy's antisocial behaviour to later aggression toward a partner than via parental dyadic aggression. An association was found between antisocial behaviour and aggression toward partners across two generations. These findings indicate that unskilled parenting and the development of antisocial behaviour can have pervasive detrimental effects on well-being that reach into adulthood.

Moving from theory to practice: developmental failure and preventive implications

Cicchetti and Schneider-Rosen (1986) presented an organisational model of child development whereby normal or successful adaptation at any given age requires the prior development of a series of interlocking social, emotional, and cognitive competencies. Thus, early adaptation is seen as promoting later adaptation, and conversely, early maladaptation is seen as promoting later maladaptation (see Sroufe 1990). We posit that antisocial behaviours interfere with the development of child competencies, and thus, when present at a given age for a sufficient duration, can initiate a cascading chain of failures that lead to negative life outcomes.

Clearly, from our discussion above, efforts early in child development to prevent the initiation and/or continuance of antisocial behaviour could have multiple benefits in preventing a wide range of individual and societal problems. As noted above and reviewed elsewhere (see Stoff *et al.* 1997), parenting practices are not only a key determinant for child antisocial behaviour but also serve as a buffer for the impact of a variety of potentially damaging contextual factors on child behaviour. Based on the scientific evidence to date, behavioural parent training is the most effective clinical intervention for child antisocial behaviour problems (Brestan and Eyberg 1998; Taylor *et al.* 1999). Parent-training programmes are a key component of the multi-setting interventions thought most likely to have the greatest impact on the prevalence of child antisocial behaviour (Greenwood *et al.* 1996; Reid and Eddy 1997). Several efficacy studies of multi-setting prevention programmes that include parent training are in progress (e.g. Hawkins *et al.* 1991; Conduct Problems Prevention Research Group 1992; Tremblay *et al.* 1995). One such study is being conducted at our centre on the LIFT programme (Linking the Interests of Families and Teachers) (Eddy *et al.* in press; Reid *et al.* 1999).

The LIFT programme

The LIFT programme is a universal preventive intervention designed for delivery within an elementary school. Because the federal government does not sponsor a national healthcare system within the United States, the earliest possible point of contact between a social service delivery system and the majority of children and families is the local public elementary school district. Contact with the majority of children and families is important in the prevention of antisocial behaviour because prediction of which specific individuals will go on to display severe antisocial behaviours is only partially accurate (Offord 1997). Further, interventions affecting an entire social group (e.g. a school) provide more leverage on individuals' behaviours. Following an ecological model, both child antisocial and child prosocial behaviour were targeted with multicomponent interventions in three settings: the home, the classroom, and the playground.

Home   Theoretically, the most important intervention component of the LIFT programme was parent training. The parent group-training meetings focused on positive reinforcement, discipline, monitoring, and problem-solving techniques that have been found to be effective with elementary school-aged children (see Eddy *et al.* in press, for more details). Sessions were offered at several times per week, and free childcare was provided. Parents who could not attend were offered sessions at home or sent written materials. In addition, the group trainer called each parent by phone between sessions to answer questions, offer encouragement, and assist with homework. Supplementary individual sessions were provided if desired to address specific family needs; however, this was relatively rare.

Classroom   Complementing the parent-training programme was the LIFT classroom programme. Classroom instructors met for 1 hour with all students within a class twice a week for 10 weeks. The first session of the week comprised lecture and role plays on a specific social or problem-solving skill, small and large group practice time, playground time, and presentation of daily rewards. The second session comprised a class meeting and problem-solving session in addition to playground and reward time. Social and problem-solving skills conducive to positive child–peer, child–teacher, and child–parent relationships were developed.

Playground   During the playground time, a version of the Good Behaviour Game (GBG) (Barrish *et al.* 1969; Dolan *et al.* 1993) was used both to reinforce prosocial, and to discourage antisocial, behaviours on the playground. Each child in the class was assigned to a group of several children, and while on the playground, could earn rewards for themselves, their group, and the entire class. Immediate rewards were distributed by playground staff, who gave children an armband and verbal praise when they were observed behaving in an overtly positive manner. Armbands from all class members were pooled in a jar at the end of recess; when the jar was full, a special treat was given to all class members. In contrast, negative behaviours were tracked on a small group chart, and groups lost points from a 'good faith' fund of points. Graduated group rewards included stickers, small prizes, and class pizza parties.

Findings of the LIFT randomised controlled trial

The LIFT study began in 1991 and comprised a longitudinal sample of three cohorts ($n = 671$) that were divided between control and intervention schools. Participants were from the same or similar neighbourhoods to the OYS and had similar demographic characteristics. A similar recruitment strategy to the OYS was used, except that all boys and girls in either the first or the fifth grades of participating public schools were invited to participate. Eighty-five per cent of those invited participated. At the 3-year follow-up, only 3% had discontinued their participation. Assessments were also similar to OYS with the addition that children were observed in the classroom and on the playground. The LIFT intervention was delivered with high fidelity in both the parent training and classroom settings. Delivering the programme in multiple ways was important in achieving the high rate of participation. Further, the majority of parents and teachers reported high levels of satisfaction with the LIFT programme. Complete details about the LIFT study are provided in Eddy *et al.* (in press) and Reid *et al.* (1999).

Immediate impact of the LIFT programme   Statistically significant differences were found between the control and intervention groups immediately following the programme on three variables predictive of later delinquency: child physical aggression toward classmates during school recess, parent aversive behaviour during family problem-solving discussions, and teacher impressions of child social skills with classmates. These differences translated into clinically significant differences between the groups. For example, prior to the programme, an average child displayed 6 aversive physical behaviours across the course of three 10-minute recess periods. Following the programme, an average child in the intervention group displayed 4.8 such behaviours, versus 6.6 in the control group. This translated to a decrease of over 1700 aversive behaviours on an average intervention classroom playground during the spring academic quarter. In addition to reducing perpetration, the LIFT intervention therefore had important benefits for children's well-being by reducing victimisation. For example, studies by Pepler and colleagues (Atlas and Pepler 1998; Pepler *et al.* 1999) have detailed the high prevalence and severe consequences of episodes of bullying in schools. Interventions such as the GBG reduce such episodes, and can be part of a school-wide antibullying programme. Interestingly, the effects of the LIFT programme were the greatest for the children who were displaying the highest rates of antisocial behaviour (Stoolmiller *et al.* 2000).

Three-year impact of the LIFT programme   Preventive effects of the LIFT programme were found in both the first- and the fifth-grade samples. Intervention first-graders were significantly less likely than those in the control group to demonstrate increases in teacher-rated inattentive, impulsive, and hyperactive behaviours over the 3-year follow-up. These behaviours are related to later delinquency (Loeber *et al.* 1995). Intervention fifth-graders were significantly delayed relative to the control group in the time to first police arrest, the time to first report by teachers that a youth was associating with deviant peers, the time to first patterned use of alcohol, and the time to first use of marijuana. These effects translated into very meaningful differences between the groups: relative to control youth, intervention youth were 2.4 times less likely to be arrested, 2.2 times less likely to associate with deviant peers, 1.8 times less likely to be involved in patterned alcohol use, and 1.5 times less likely to have used marijuana. Early police arrest (i.e. before age 14), association with deviant peers, and early substance use are strongly correlated with serious delinquency during the adolescent years (Dishion *et al.* 1995)

Discussion

The design of the LIFT programme was based on the findings of OYS and other studies, with the intent of integrating theoretically sound and practically promising preventive intervention techniques into a package that could easily and inexpensively be integrated into the day-to-day activities of an elementary school. The parent, classroom, and playground components were well liked by both parents and teachers, intervention fidelity can be maintained across a wide spectrum of staff training and experience, and high participation rates can be achieved. Under the conditions of a tightly controlled randomised evaluation, the LIFT programme has been demonstrated to impact the conduct problems that precede delinquent behaviour during elementary school and delinquent and other problem behaviours during adolescence. Further, this impact appeared to be strongest for the children who exhibited the highest rates of problem behaviours.

As developmental and clinical researchers, we are quite aware of the difficulties in changing antisocial behaviour patterns. In fact, this awareness was one of the reasons that we as a research group began to develop not only preventive work, but also intensive individualised residential interventions such as Multi-dimensional Treatment Foster Care (Chamberlain and Reid 1998). From this base of experience, the impact of the LIFT programme on high-rate children has been quite surprising to us. On reflection, there are several possible reasons for this effect. First, children with extreme behaviour problems tend to live in a social world that provides a rich array of reinforcers for their antisocial behaviours and few reinforcers for their positive behaviours. In targeting an entire school class in the LIFT programme, rather than individual children within a class, the density of reinforcement for positive behaviours for each of the individuals within the class became much higher, which in turn provided high-rate children with the opportunity to develop a new set of behaviours. This would simply not be possible unless the majority of children and adults in a child's world were working together to create a mutually beneficial positive environment. In effect, each individual within the class becomes a treatment agent.

Second, the relatively slight changes in rates of aversive physical behaviour on the playground actually led to rather large changes in overall exposure to risk (i.e. 1700 less physically aversive events on the playground). This lessening of cumulative exposure to noxious social interactions may have the largest payoffs for the most behaviourally vulnerable children.

We propose that interventions such as the GBG or even child problem-solving and social-skills training have their most powerful effects on a given social milieu as a whole, which in turn has effects on individuals within the milieu, rather than vice versa. Unfortunately, if new children who enter the milieu have well-developed repertoires of problem behaviours, the new pattern that is developed may be ruled by coercion (Patterson 1982), particularly in less structured settings such as the playground. It is not uncommon for many of the classmates of a child, and certainly his or her teacher, to change on a yearly basis. On the other hand, because parents were also involved in the LIFT programme, we hypothesised that we would find a lasting impact of the intervention on children and their families, and this would lead to various positive child outcomes such as lower rates of involvement with deviant peers and lower arrest rates. To date, we have found support for this hypothesis. Whether the LIFT programme ultimately does impact the total frequency and content of delinquent behaviour, including violence, throughout adolescence and into young adulthood remains under investigation. Within the next 3 years, all participants in the fifth-grade sample will reach the age of 19; therefore, information on this important issue is forthcoming.

Findings from the OYS confirmed the theoretical expectations and results of prior studies suggesting that antisocial behaviour in childhood is associated with key developmental failures and has very detrimental outcomes for the well-being of the child. These detrimental effects also diminish the well-being of others in their lives, with consequences that reach into adulthood. The OYS findings also confirmed the importance of the role of parenting practices as being implicated in the development of antisocial behaviour in childhood. The multipronged LIFT intervention was designed to improve parenting practices as well as to improve peer interactions and school adjustment. Findings from the LIFT programme provide great promise that such interventions can make a meaningful and long-lasting improvement in the well-being both of the children with antisocial behaviour problems and their victims, by reducing the levels of antisocial behaviours. Whereas this preventive work is

promising, changing antisocial behaviour patterns is very difficult. Low-intensity interventions such as the LIFT programme
may change the trajectories of some children who would otherwise have more serious behaviour problems; however, a full
range of interventions is needed if the problems of childhood
antisocial behaviour, delinquency, and violence are to be
addressed adequately. We have investigated the impact of interventions based on the coercion model with high-rate juvenile
offenders and have found, even with these individuals, positive
and clinically significant impacts (e.g. Chamberlain and Reid
1998). Overall, our work has reaffirmed the idea that interventions must address child behaviours within the social arenas of
their lives. If the majority of children and adults in a child's
world are working together to create a mutually beneficial,
positive environment, change can and often does occur. Taken
together with promising interventions developed for different
phases of the life span, such as home visiting for at-risk pregnant
mothers (Olds *et al.* 1998) and pre-school interventions
(Webster-Stratton 1998), two decades of intensive research on
these topics appear to be culminating in well-designed programmes that can make a real difference for family well-being.

Acknowledgements

The authors would like to thank the following for permission
to reproduce published material: American Psychological
Association, *Developmental Psychology* (Fig. 10.2).

Support for the Oregon Youth Study was provided by Grant
MH 37940 from the Prevention, Early Intervention, and
Epidemiology Branch (NIMH (National Institute of Mental
Health), US PHS (Public Health Service)). Support for the LIFT
Study was provided by Grant MH 54248 from the Prevention
and Behavioral Medicine Research Branch, Division of
Epidemiology and Services Research (NIMH, US PHS). Additional
support was provided by Grant MH 46690 from the Prevention
Early Intervention, and Epidemiology Branch (NIMH, US PHS);
Grant MH 50259 Prevention, Early Intervention, and
Epidemiology Branch (NIMH, US PHS).

References

Atlas, R. S. and Pepler, D. J. (1998). Observations of bullying in the classroom. *Journal of Educational Research*, **92**, 86–99.

Barrish, H. H., Saunders, M., and Wolf, M. M. (1969). Good behaviour game: effects of individual contingencies for group consequences on disruptive behavior in a classroom. *Journal of Applied Behavior Analysis*, **2**, 119–24.

Brestan, E. V. and Eyberg, S. M. (1998). Effective psychosocial treatments of conduct-disordered children and adolescents: 29 years, 82 studies, and 5,272 kids. *Journal of Clinical Child Psychology*, **27**, 180–9.

Capaldi, D. M., Chamberlain, P., Fetrow, R. A., and Wilson, J. (1997). Conducting ecologically valid prevention research: recruiting and retaining a 'whole village' in multimethod, multiagent studies. *American Journal of Community Psychology*, **25**, 471–92.

Capaldi, D. M. and Clark, S. (1998). Prospective family predictors of aggression toward female partners for at-risk young men. *Developmental Psychology*, **34**, 1175–88.

Capaldi, D. M. and Patterson, G. R. (1991). Relation of parental transitions to boys' adjustment problems: I. a linear hypothesis; II. mothers at risk for transitions and unskilled parenting. *Developmental Psychology*, **27**, 489–504.

Capaldi, D. M. and Stoolmiller, M. (1999). Co-occurrence of conduct problems and depressive symptoms in early adolescent boys: III. prediction to young-adult adjustment. *Development and Psychopathology*, **11**, 59–84.

Chamberlain, P. and Reid, J. (1998). Comparison of two community alternatives to incarceration for chronic juvenile offenders. *Journal of Consulting and Clinical Psychology*, **6**, 624–33.

Cherlin, A. J., Furstenberg, F. F., Jr, Chase-Lansdale, P. L., *et al.* (1991). Longitudinal studies of effects of divorce on children in Great Britain and the United States. *Science*, **252**, 1386–9.

Cicchetti, D. and Schneider-Rosen, K. (1986). An organizational approach to childhood depression. In M. Rutter, C. E. Izard, and P. B. Read (eds.), *Depression in young people: developmental and clinical perspectives*, pp. 71–134. New York, Guilford.

Cohen, L. H., Burt, C. E., and Bjorck, J. P. (1987). Life stress and adjustment: effects of life events experienced by young adolescents and their parents. *Developmental Psychology*, **23**, 583–92.

Conduct Problems Prevention Research Group (1992). A developmental and clinical model for prevention of conduct disorders: the FAST Track program. *Development and Psychopathology*, **4**, 509–27.

DeBaryshe, B. D., Patterson, G. R., and Capaldi, D. M. (1993). A performance model for academic achievement in early adolescent boys. *Developmental Psychology*, **29**, 795–804.

Dishion, T. J., French, D. C., and Patterson, G. R. (1995). The development and ecology of antisocial behavior. In D. Cicchetti and D. J. Cohen (eds.), *Developmental psychopathology. Vol. 2: risk, disorder, and adaptation*, pp. 421–71. New York, Wiley.

Dishion, T. J., Patterson, G. R., Stoolmiller, M., and Skinner, M. L. (1991). Family, school, and behavioral antecedents to early adolescent involvement with antisocial peers. *Developmental Psychology*, **27**, 172–80.

Dolan, L. J., Kellam, S. G., Brown, C. H., *et al.* (1993). The short-term impact of two classroom-based preventive interventions on aggressive and shy behaviors and poor achievement. *Journal of Applied Developmental Psychology*, **14**, 317–45.

Eddy, J. M., Reid, J. B., and Fetrow, R. A. (in press). An elementary-school based prevention program targeting modifiable antecedents of youth delinquency and violence: Linking the Interests of Families and Teachers (LIFT). *Journal of Emotional and Behavioral Disorders.*

Elliott, D. S., Huizinga, D., and Ageton, S. S. (1985). *Explaining delinquency and drug use.* Beverly Hills, CA, Sage.

Farrington, D. P. (1979). Longitudinal research on crime and delinquency. In N. Morris and M. Tonry (eds.), *Crime and justice: a longitudinal review of research. Vol. 1*, pp. 289–348. Chicago, University of Chicago Press.

Forgatch, M. S. (1991). The clinical science vortex: developing a theory for antisocial behavior. In D. J. Pepler and K. H. Rubin (eds.), *The development and treatment of childhood aggression*, pp. 291–315. Hillsdale, NJ, Erlbaum.

Forgatch, M. S. and Patterson, G. R. (1989). *Parents and adolescents living together. Part 2: family problem solving.* Eugene, OR, Castalia.

Forgatch, M. S., Patterson, G. R., and Ray, J. A. (1996). Divorce and boys' adjustment problems: two paths with a single model. In E. M. Hetherington (ed.), *Stress, coping, and resiliency in children and the family*, pp. 67–105. Hillsdale, NJ, Erlbaum.

Forgatch, M. S., Patterson, G. R., and Skinner, M. L. (1988). A mediational model for the effect of divorce on antisocial behavior in boys. In E. M. Hetherington and J. D. Aresteh (eds.), *Impact of divorce, single parenting, and step-parenting on children*, pp. 135–54. Hillsdale, NJ, Erlbaum.

Freeman, R. B. (1983). Crime and unemployment. In J. Q. Wilson (ed.), *Crime and public policy*, pp. 89–106. San Francisco, ICS.

Gersten, J. C., Langner, T. S., Eisenberg, J. G., and Simcha-Fagan, O. (1977). An evaluation of the etiological role of stressful life-change events in psychological disorders. *Journal of Health and Social Behavior*, **18**, 228–44.

Greenwood, P. W., Model, K. E., Rydell, C. P., and Chiesa, J. (1996). *Diverting children from a life of crime: measuring costs and benefits* (Report No. MR-699.0-UCB/RC/IF). Berkeley, RAND Corporation.

Hawkins, J. D., Von Cleve, E., and Catalano, R. F. (1991). Reducing early childhood aggression: results of a primary prevention program. *Journal of the American Academy of Child and Adolescent Psychiatry*, **30**, 208–17.

Hetherington, E. M., Cox, M., and Cox, R. (1979). Family interaction and the social, emotional, and cognitive development of children following divorce. In V. Vaughn and T. Brazelton (eds.), *The family: setting priorities*, pp. 89–128. New York, Science and Medicine.

Hetherington, E. M., Cox, M., and Cox, R. (1981). Effects of divorce on parents and children. In M. Lamb (ed.), *Nontraditional families*, pp. 233–87. Hillsdale, NJ, Erlbaum.

Kohlberg, L., Ricks, D., and Snarey, J. (1984). Childhood development as a predictor of adaptation in adulthood. *Genetic Psychology Monographs*, **110**, 91–172.

Loeber, R., Green, S. M., Keenan, K., and Lahey, B. B. (1995). Which boys will fare worse? Early predictors of the onset of conduct disorder in a six-year longitudinal study. *Journal of the American Academy of Child and Adolescent Psychiatry*, **34**, 499–509.

Offord, D. R. (1997). Bridging development, prevention, and policy. In D. Stoff, J. Breiling, and J. Maser (eds.), *Handbook of antisocial behavior*, pp. 357–64. New York, Wiley.

Offord, D. R., Boyle, M. C., and Racine, Y. A. (1991). The epidemiology of antisocial behavior in childhood and adolescence. In D. J. Pepler and K. H. Rubin (eds.), *The development and treatment of childhood aggression*, pp. 31–54. Hillsdale, NJ, Erlbaum.

Olds, D., Pettitt, L. M., Robinson, J., *et al.* (1998). Reducing risks for antisocial behavior with a program of prenatal and early childhood home visitation. *Journal of Community Psychology*, **26**, 65–83.

Patterson, G. R. (1982). *Coercive family process.* Eugene, OR, Castalia.

Patterson, G. R. (1986). Performance models for antisocial boys. *American Psychologist*, **41**, 432–44.

Patterson, G. R., Capaldi, D. M., and Bank, L. (1991). An early starter model predicting delinquency. In D. J. Pepler and K. H. Rubin (eds.), *The development and treatment of childhood aggression*, pp. 139–68. Hillsdale, NJ, Erlbaum.

Patterson, G. R. and Forgatch, M. S. (1995). Predicting future clinical adjustment from treatment outcome and process variables. *Psychological Assessment*, **7**, 275–85.

Patterson, G. R., Reid, J. B., and Dishion, T. J. (1992). *A social learning approach. IV. Antisocial boys.* Eugene, OR, Castalia.

Pepler, D., Craig, W. M., and O'Connell, P. (1999). Understanding bullying from a dynamic systems perspective. In A. Slater and D. Muir (eds.), *The Blackwell reader in development psychology*, pp. 440–51. Malden, MA, Blackwell.

Ramsey, E., Patterson, G. R., and Walker, H. M. (1990). Generalization of the antisocial trait from home to school settings. *Journal of Applied Developmental Psychology*, **11**, 209–23.

Reid, J. B. and Eddy, J. M. (1997). The prevention of antisocial behavior: some considerations in the search for effective interventions. In D. M. Stoff, J. Breiling, and J. D. Maser (eds.), *Handbook of antisocial behavior*, pp. 343–56. New York, Wiley.

Reid, J. B., Eddy, J. M., Fetrow, R. A., and Stoolmiller, M. (1999). Description and immediate impacts of a preventative intervention for conduct problems. *American Journal of Community Psychology*, **24**, 483–517.

Reiss, A. J. (1986). Co-offender influences on criminal careers. In A. Blumstein, J. Cohen, J. Roth, and C. Visher (eds.), *Criminal careers and career criminals*, pp. 121–59. Washington, DC, National Academy Press.

Rutter, M. and Giller, H. (1983). *Juvenile delinquency: trends and perspectives*. Middlesex, Penguin.

Santrock, J. W. (1972). Relation of type and onset of father absence to cognitive development. *Child Development*, **43**, 455–69.

Snyder, J. J. (1991). Discipline as a mediator of the impact of maternal stress and mood on child conduct problems. *Development and Psychopathology*, **3**, 263–76.

Sroufe, L. A. (1990). Considering normal and abnormal together: the essence of developmental psychopathology. *Development and Psychopathology*, **2**, 335–47.

Stoff, D. M., Breiling, J., and Maser, J. D. (eds.) (1997). *Handbook of antisocial behavior*. New York, Wiley.

Stoolmiller, M. (1994). Antisocial behavior, delinquent peer association, and unsupervised wandering for boys: growth and change from childhood to early adolescence. *Multivariate Behavioral Research*, **29**, 263–88.

Stoolmiller, M., Duncan, T. E., and Patterson, G. R. (1995). Predictors of change in antisocial behavior during elementary school for boys. In R. H. Hoyle (ed.), *Structural equation modeling: concepts, issues, and applications*, pp. 236–53. Newbury Park, CA, Sage.

Stoolmiller, M., Eddy, J. M., and Reid, J. B. (2000). Detecting and describing preventative intervention effects in a universally school-based randomized trail targeting delinquent and violent behavior. *Journal of Consulting and Clinical Psychology*, **2**, 269–306.

Taylor, T. K., Eddy, J. M., and Biglan, A. (1999). Interpersonal skills training to reduce aggressive and delinquent behavior: limited evidence and the need for an evidence-based system of care. *Clinical Child and Family Psychology Review*, **2**, 169–82.

Tooliatos, J. and Lindholm, B. W. (1980). Teachers' perceptions of behavior problems in children from intact, single parent, and step-parent families. *Psychology in the Schools*, **17**, 264–9.

Tremblay, R. E., Japel, C., Perusse, D., *et al.* (1999). The search for the age of 'onset' of physical aggression: Rousseau and Bandura revisited. *Criminal Behavior and Mental Health*, **9**, 8–13.

Tremblay, R. E., Pagani-Kurtz, L., Masse, L. C., *et al.* (1995). A bimodal preventive intervention for disruptive kindergarten boys: its impact through mid-adolescence. *Journal of Consulting and Clinical Psychology*, **63**, 560–8.

Wallerstein, J. S. and Kelly, J. B. (1980). *Surviving the breakup: how children and parents cope with divorce*. New York, Basic Books.

Webster-Stratton, C. (1998). Preventing conduct problems in Head Start children: strengthening parenting competencies. *Journal of Consulting and Clinical Psychology*, **66**, 715–30.

Wilson, H. (1987). Parental supervision re-examined. *British Journal of Criminology*, **27**, 215–301.

11

Messages from the research

Ann Buchanan

*'Our challenge now is to be conscious of what we have learned, to
monitor our expanding knowledge base and to continually pull
in new insights, new experiences which contribute to our ability
to understand . . . And then our commitment must be to base our
policies and our program decisions and budget allocations on
that which we have learned.'* Cohn 1992, p. xv

The task of this final chapter is to bring together the central
messages that have emerged from the preceding chapters. The
increasing volume of research in this field has taken us up the
slopes of a hill; ahead is the peak; once there all will be clear. The
peak, however, proves to be yet another ridge beyond which
there is a further top to climb. As each ridge is past, a whole new
vista presents. Ann Cohn, quoted above, was speaking in 1992.
The focus at that time was on breaking the cycle of child abuse.
Child abuse was, and remains, one of the greatest threats to a
child's well-being. In the UK and US, throughout the 1970s,
1980s, and early 1990s, a huge industry developed to protect
children. Then, in the UK, came *Child protection: messages from
research* (Department of Health 1995). This summarised over 20
research studies into the workings of procedures to protect
children. The key message was that, although children in
dangerous situations should be protected, the focus of intervention should change to improving the emotional well-being of
much larger numbers of children damaged by living in families 'low
in warmth and high in criticism'.

Long-term problems occur when the parenting style fails to compensate for the inevitable deficiencies that become manifest in the course of 20 years or so it takes to bring up a child. During this period, occasional neglect, unnecessary or severe punishment or some form of family discord can be expected . . . if parenting is entirely negative, it will be damaging . . . In families low on warmth and high on criticism, negative incidents accumulate as if to remind a child that he or she is unloved. (Department of Health 1995, p. 19.)

Studies from the US, in particular the early studies by Patterson, outlined by Gardner and Ward in Chapter 5, added fuel to the concept that the key agent to promote children's well-being was the parent(s). This body of research showed that children's behaviour improved if parents adopted a less 'coercive' style. In a sense the long-standing 'anti-smacking' campaign to clarify the law in England and Wales on the traditional defence of 'reasonable chastisement', which led to the consultation paper (Department of Health 2000), was also about encouraging more positive methods of parental discipline.

As is seen in Chapter 5, the particular concern was the association between 'coercive' or punitive style parenting and conduct disorders. Concerns about youth crime, the rise in the numbers of children with psychosocial disorders (Rutter and Smith 1995), and the long-term consequences of such disorders suggested that any intervention, activity, or service that prevented maladjustment, delay, or disorder (Simeonsson 1994) would have the reciprocal benefit of promoting a child's development, adaptation, or functioning. That was the starting point of this book.

What is emotional well-being?

Very quickly this rather limited vision was challenged. In Chapter 2 a much wider public health view of well-being emerges. Health is not just the absence of disease, or functionality and the ability to cope. The WHO definition suggests that health is a state of complete physical, mental, and social well-being, not merely the absence of disease. The presence or absence of health is determined by the subjective assessment of the individual concerned, not by the objective assessment of others.

Other contributors also challenge the rather limited vision presented in Chapter 1. For example Gardner and Ward suggest that children's well-being should be seen as more than merely the absence of behavioural problems.

Stewart-Brown gives us a much wider vision of emotional well-being:

a holistic, subjective state which is present when a range of feelings, among them energy, confidence, openness, enjoyment, happiness, calm, and caring, are combined and balanced. (see page 32)

Following on from these ideas, Wells argues in Chapter 8 that there is a need for new, valid, and reliable measures of emotional well-being in children.

From Wells' review, and those of other contributors, comes the idea that well-being is something different from the absence of problems, something more than a lack of depression, something more than happiness. Into the model comes confidence, empathy, prosocial behaviour, creativity, and a sense of achievement. This global sense of well-being incorporates many of the existing measures used to assess different components of well-being in children; for example scales to measure strengths/difficulties, self-esteem, self-efficacy, locus of control, empathy; but none of these scales appear to capture the essence of global emotional well-being.

If this is true, there is a further peak to climb. Research will be needed to develop scales to measure global emotional well-being in children; prevalence studies; studies on risk and protective factors associated with well-being; experimental studies to test the effectiveness of interventions to promote well-being; longitudinal studies to trace outcomes from childhood to adult life.

Subjective well-being

In trying to define emotional well-being in children, it may be profitable to look more closely at the literature on subjective well-being (SWB) in adults. Over the years, the concept of SWB has changed (Diener *et al.* 1999). Wilson in 1967 found that 'happy' people were young, healthy, well-educated, well-paid, religious, married, with high job morale, of either sex, and of any level of intelligence. Many of Wilson's conclusions were overturned. In particular his conclusion that youth and modest aspirations are essential prerequisites to SWB no longer stands. By 1999 the concept of SWB had moved beyond measuring ' happiness' to include a more rational response. SWB is now viewed as a broad category of phenomena that include people's emotional responses (affect), as well as satisfaction in different domains of their lives, and more global judgements of life satisfaction. Andrews and Robinson (1991) consider measures of life satisfaction as the 'bottom-line' calculation of what a person wanted versus what they feel they have achieved. Measures of life satisfaction are related not only to feelings about family, relationships, and work, but to non-work activities and leisure.

Michalos (1985) has advanced the multiple discrepancy theory of life satisfaction whereby individuals compare themselves to multiple standards including other people, past conditions, aspirations and ideal levels of satisfaction, needs, and goals. Satisfaction judgements are then based on discrepancies between current conditions and these standards.

Although personality is one of the strongest and most consistent predictors of subjective well-being, Diener *et al.*'s conclusions reflect those of Rutter (1999) in relation to child psychopathology discussed in Chapter 1; biology, or genes, are only part of the story. When it comes to levels of subjective well-being, personality interacts with situations and the environment (Diener *et al.* 1999).

In current research on SWB, Austin and Vancouver (1996) also examine 'goals': what people are trying to do in life and how well they are succeeding. Life satisfaction, of course, is related to whether the goals chosen are obtainable.

Diener *et al.* (1999, p. 295) conclude that the person with SWB:

Is blessed with a positive temperament, tends to look on the bright side of things, and does not ruminate excessively about bad events, and is living in a economically developed society, has social confidants, and possesses adequate resources for making progress toward valued goals.

Is this emotional well-being? Perhaps, but even this is not the whole story. Contributors to this book indicate that a definition of emotional well-being goes beyond the above. It is possible to imagine a very 'satisfied' and 'successful' young person who meets the criteria, but obtains his sense of well-being from anti-social activities. A definition of emotional well-being in children needs to include an element that indicates prosocial values.

Well-being is influenced by events happening in different domains of the child's life

Andrews and Robinson (1991) note that life satisfaction is related to personal calculations about how well things are going in different domains of life. In this publication, a key message is that children's emotional well-being, the wider concept described above, is not something that just happens at home. There is considerable agreement that children's well-being has to be seen in relation to social contexts in which the children and their families operate. A simplified version of Bronfenbrenner's (1979) interacting 'ecological framework' was outlined in Chapter 1. Risk and protective factors were present in each of the domains, the 'person', 'the family', 'the school', and the 'wider world'. No judgement was made about the relative strengths of each domain.

Stewart-Brown's model was a little different. She places healthy parenting and social well-being in the home at the centre of her model, with social well-being in communities and workplace and public policy impacting on this and radiating out into the child's well-being in adolescence and adulthood.

Capaldi and Eddy's model from the Oregon Social Learning Centre recognises that 'all families operate within a larger con-text of factors that affect internal family process, either in a sup-portive or detrimental fashion'. They noted the impact of stress events, education and occupation, child temperament, school, substance abuse, divorce, and deviant peers on parenting effec-tiveness, but in their model Capaldi and Eddy posit that many of the effects of contextual variables on antisocial behaviour are mediated through family and *peer process variables*.

Intervening in the different domains for greater impact

Since well-being is influenced by happenings in different domains of a child's life, it makes sense that interventions to promote his or her well-being can take place in different domains in the child's life (home, school, community) or in multi-domains. Wells, in Chapter 8, demonstrates in her systematic review that school-based interventions can have a significant impact on the mental health of the general population of children. Baillie, Sylva, and Evans in Chapter 7 show the value of the home–school link.

The LIFT programme described in Chapter 10 also has a parent–classroom–playground link. Although theoretically the most important intervention component of the LIFT programme is parent-training, it is strongly complemented by the classroom and playground elements. Capaldi and Eddy found statistically significant differences between the intervention and control groups, not only in the short term but *3 years* after the original interventions.

Wells, in her systematic review, also found that school-based approaches were more effective if they were complementary to other areas of the children's lives. She found that there was evidence to support the effectiveness of a comprehensive approach involving the whole school and community.

The importance of interdisciplinary research

Since multi-domain interventions to promote children's well-being may be more effective than single-system approaches, the corollary is that *interdisciplinary* research will be needed to assess the impact of different approaches. The *raison d'être* of The Centre for Research for Parenting and Children, the group that gave birth to this book, rests in the belief that advances in research will arise from such a coming together.

Bringing the contributors to this book together, however, highlights the different responsibilities, the different priorities of the different professions, and also the different research traditions within the different disciplines. Stewart-Brown's role is to investigate how the public health of all children can be promoted. Her research tradition is epidemiology. Baillie, Sylva, and Evans' priority, coming from an educational studies department, is research into methods of improving the educational attainments of children. Grimshaw, on the other hand, came originally from the multidisciplinary Birmingham-based cultural studies tradition, influenced by Stuart Hall. Gardner and Ward, and Capaldi and Eddy, come from a clinical psychological and developmental tradition. Their training is based on rigorous experimental research. Hunt, specialising in socio-legal studies, has focused on quantitative and qualitative descriptive research that informs the legal process.

Each discipline has a contribution to make. An important message from this book is that the researchers contributing to it, often using very different research methods and very different research samples, come together like pieces of a jigsaw puzzle to present a more coherent picture of the whole.

Interventions at different levels

A further message from this book is that efforts to promote the emotional well-being of children need to be exerted at different levels. *At a population* level achievements in improving the well-being of the whole child population may well result in fewer children with serious problems (Stewart-Brown 1998). Similarly, population approaches in schools are likely to reduce the numbers of children who are traumatised by bullying, for example. Nevertheless there will remain some seriously disturbed young people who *individually* will need special care from psychologists, social workers, and even the law.

Interventions need to improve on natural improvements

In descriptive research, studies where there are no controls, it is tempting to credit positive outcomes to the effect of the intervention. In Chapter 3, we see that between ages 7 and 11 around 50% of children with emotional and/or behavioural problems 'recover' and similarly 50% recover between 11 and 16. To be 'effective', interventions must improve on the natural recovery rate that children will achieve in the course of growing up. Further randomised controlled trials are needed if progress is to be made on this front. As noted in Chapter 1, the UK lags behind the US in this respect.

The major dilemma is that some well-meaning interventions currently being implemented may inadvertently harm. In the US, before funding a project most funders require a commitment to evaluate. In the UK funders are curiously reluctant to spend money on anything more than a simple evaluation of a project. These simple evaluations will tell them very little about cost-effectiveness. Of the evaluations that have been undertaken in the UK, as Jane Wells notes in Chapter 8, very few meet the necessary standards to draw safe conclusions.

Longitudinal studies, as seen in Chapter 3, also indicate that well-being needs to be measured over time. Short-term problems in relation to well-being may not predict long-term outcomes. Into the equation also come the developmental forces of child-hood, suggesting the ages when lack of well-being is more or less likely. In addition, research into emotional and behavioural problems shows that boys and girls have different critical times and different pathways from childhood into adult life (Buchanan and Ten Brinke 1998).

In social programmes, the 'pill' has to be made palatable

The scientific tradition in reporting research for peer reviewed journals can make some reporting of social interventions sound mechanistic: all that needs to be done is 'to prescribe the pill' – the social intervention. As those who have been involved in successful programmes know, there is much more to it. Families do not become involved in social interventions unless there is an element of trust and a belief that what is being offered is what they want and will be likely to improve their situation (Buchanan 1999). Outsiders may believe that a mother/father needs to take part in a parenting programme, but parents whose children are having difficulties will be very reluctant to attend a parenting programme: firstly, they may believe that this tantamount to admitting that they have problems; secondly, they may be worried that the programme providers will report them to social services. Finally, if parents are not enjoying parenting, it may be the last way they wish to spend any spare time they have.

Grimshaw reminds us in Chapter 6 that, at the end of the day, most parents have the choice about whether or not to take part in a parenting programme. Consequent on this, it is important for those planning to use validated programmes to check carefully how the programme is presented to families. How many parents were approached and decided not to take part? What incentives were offered to parents to take part? Were those who took part parents with parenting difficulties, or parents who were already parenting effectively and may not have needed help? How many parents started to attend and then dropped out?

Researchers who have developed well-validated programmes worry about implementing them with 'integrity' (Webster-Stratton 1998). A programme provider cannot expect to obtain the same results if the 'ethos' surrounding a programme is different to that intended, if considerable changes have been made, or if only part of the programme is provided.

When the state becomes the public parent

In the 1970s there was a belief that children from malfunctioning families, particularly where there was abuse or neglect, could be 'rescued' to a better life in public care. Studies in the UK and elsewhere (Department of Health 1991; Barth *et al.* 1994) are testament that this is very difficult to achieve. Gibbons *et al.* (1995) summarise the conclusions from their study:

We could find no evidence that children who were legally protected . . . did significantly better. Nor do those removed from their abusers and placed in new permanent or long term- families have significantly better outcomes than those who remained with their original carers. (Quoted on p. 50, Department of Health 1995.)

A further concern in the UK is the number of inquiries relating to abuse while in the care system (Warner Report 1992). As noted earlier, in England and Wales the anxieties that large numbers of children were unnecessarily going through child protection procedures led to pressures to refocus social services away from protective work and towards more family support.

In the US there has been a similar pattern of concern:

There has been an urgent need in the United States for a comprehensive family policy that supports rather than controls caregivers and for an improvement in general social services ... (this) would assist families to respond in more nurturing ways to children's needs while not eliminating the necessity for protective services. (Hutchison 1994, p. 23.)

In social policy research, there is a longstanding tradition of exploring the 'unintended consequences' of policy change. Joan Hunt's study on the effects of delay in court proceedings where it was unlikely that children could safely return to live with their parents, is such a study. Under the Children Act 1989 in England and Wales, when a court determines any question with respect to the upbringing of a child:

... the child's welfare shall be the court's paramount consideration. (Children Act 1989, Section 1(a).)

In these extreme cases, the law is intended as the ultimate guardian of the child's well-being. As Hunt notes, it is an uncomfortable thought that actions intended to promote the child's welfare inadvertently have had the reverse effect. Her study is an important reminder that without monitoring our legal processes we cannot be sure that outcomes will be those intended.

Intergenerational watch

A message from Chapter 3, 'In and out of behavioural problems', and from the Capaldi and Eddy chapter, is that outcomes for children may not be apparent in the short term. It is only by tracking groups of children in the long term, from childhood into adolescence, to adulthood, and into the next generation, that a picture emerges of how to promote well-being. In the UK the national birth cohort studies have provided a wealth of information. There are very few longitudinal studies that take us into the next generation. In the UK, the 1991 sweep of the National

Child Development Study includes a sample of cohort members' children. The Oregon Youth Study reported in Chapter 10 is remarkable in that, although only just over 200 boys were involved, very detailed assessments have been taken at every stage. In the teenage years the boys' current partners were also interviewed and videoed. A vivid picture emerges of parent anti-social behaviour leading to child antisocial behaviour leading to adolescent aggression to partners.

In the UK, a new sweep of both the National Child Development Study and the 1970 Bristol cohort is currently being undertaken, and it is planned that a new birth cohort study will commence in 2001.

Although longitudinal studies have their own problems (see Chapter 3), the possibility of finding out what happens in the next generation is an exciting one and promises to be hugely informative.

Getting inside children's heads

It is ironic that, for so long, there was a reluctance to listen to the one group of people who are 'experts' on their situation – the young people themselves, and it is perhaps from them that the strongest message in this book comes. Given the opportunity they have important things to say. Parenting style affects how they feel about themselves; factors at school and in the wider world, such as issues relating to the changing roles of men and women, all impinge.

There are other issues that are less well evidenced in research. For example, the strongly protective role of an 'involved' father emerges. This involved father, as we saw, is protective against alienation from school, depression and suicidal behaviour, and being in trouble with the police. The young people also highlight the destructive effects on fragile adolescent self-esteem of teachers at school who make them feel silly if they ask a question; the consequences, not only of bullying and violence at school, but also of bullying policies that do not work. More poignant still are the depressed and suicidal young people who have no one to talk to.

The strong associations seen in Chapter 4 with a range of positive outcomes suggest that, as a construct, 'Can-do' may be worth exploring further.

- I feel happy and confident about myself.
- There are exciting opportunities for me.
- I get on with my work / I set myself high standards.

If we add to this some measure of prosocial behaviour or aspiration, are these the characteristics of a child with emotional well-being? Happiness and confidence; positive views about the future, and sufficient get-up-and-go energy to achieve goals. They appear to be. The young people have a message. If we want to promote their psychological health, we need their expertise. As young people help us enter their private world, a clearer vision will emerge of what really matters to them, and a clear picture of what needs to change in order to promote their well-being will become apparent.

References

Andrews, F. M. and Robinson, J. P. (1991). Measures of subjective well-being. In J. P. Robinson, R. Shaver, and L. S. Wrightsman (eds.), *Measure of personality and social psychological attitudes.* San Diego, Academic, pp. 61–114.

Austin, J. T. and Vancouver, J. F. (1996). Goal constructs in psychology: structure, process and content. *Psychological Bulletin.* **120**, 338–75.

Barth, R., Berrick, J., and Gilbert, N. (eds.) (1994). *Child welfare research review.* New York, Columbia University Press.

Bronfenbrenner, U. (1979). *The ecology of human development: experiments by nature and design.* Cambridge, MA, Harvard University Press.

Buchanan, A. (1999). *What works for troubled children? Family support for children with emotional and behavioural problems.* London, Barnardo's.

Buchanan, A., Ten Brinke, J-A., and Flouri, E. (forthcoming). Emotional and behavioural problems in childhood and depression in adult life. Risk and protective clusters at age 7 associated with continuity and discontinuity.

Buchanan, A. and Ten-Brinke J-A. (1998) *'Recovery' from emotional and behavioural problems.* Report to NHS Executive Anglia and Oxford.

Cohn, A. (1992). Foreword: Child abuse prevention. In D. Willis, E.

242 *Promoting children's emotional well-being*

Holden, and M. Rosenberg, *Prevention of child maltreatment*. New York, Wiley.

Department of Health (1991). *Patterns and outcomes in child placement*. London, HMSO.

Department of Health (1995). *Child protection: messages from research*. London, HMSO.

Department of Health (2000). *Protecting children, supporting parents: a consultation document on the physical punishment of children*. London, Department of Health.

Diener, E., Suh, E. M., Lucas, R. E., and Smith, H. L. (1999). Subjective well-being: three decades of progress. *Psychological Bulletin, American Psychological Association*, **125**(2), 276–302.

Gibbons, J., Gallagher, B., Bell, C., and Gordon, D. (1995) *Development after physical abuse in early childhood: a follow-up study of children on child protection registers*. London, HMSO.

Hutchison, E. (1994). Defining child abuse and neglect. In R. Barth, J. Berrick, and N. Gilbert (eds.), *Child welfare research review*. New York, Columbia University Press, pp. 5–27.

Michalos, A. C. (1985). Multiple Discrepancies Theory (MDT). *Social Indicators Research*, **16**, 347–413.

Rutter, M. (1999). Psychosocial adversity and child psychopathology. *British Journal of Psychiatry* **174**, 480–493

Rutter, M. and Smith, D. (eds.) (1995). *Psychosocial disorders in young people: trends and their causes*. Chichester, Wiley.

Simeonsson, R. (1994). Promoting childrens' health, education and well-being. In R. Simeonsson (ed.), *Risk, resilience and prevention: promotion of the well-being of children*. Baltimore, Brookes, pp. 3–12.

Stewart-Brown, S. (1998). Public health implications of childhood behaviour problems and parenting programmes. In. A. Buchanan and B. L. Hudson (eds.), *Parenting, schooling and children's behaviour*. Aldershot, Ashgate, pp. 21–33.

Warner Report (1992). *Choosing with care – The report of the Committee of Inquiry into the selection, development and management of staff in children's homes*. London, HMSO.

Webster-Stratton, C. (1998). Adopting and implementing empirically supported interventions: a recipe for success. In A. Buchanan and B. L. Hudson (eds.), *Parenting, schooling and children's behaviour*. Aldershot, Ashgate, pp. 127–60.

Wilson, W. (1967). Correlates of avowed happiness. *Psychological Bulletin*, **67**, 294–306.

Index

256 *Index*